Evidence-Based Treatment Guidelines for Treating Injured Workers

Editors

ANDREW S. FRIEDMAN
GARY M. FRANKLIN

PHYSICAL MEDICINE AND REHABILITATION CLINICS OF NORTH AMERICA

www.pmr.theclinics.com

Consulting Editor
GREGORY T. CARTER

August 2015 • Volume 26 • Number 3

ELSEVIER

1600 John F. Kennedy Boulevard • Suite 1800 • Philadelphia, Pennsylvania, 19103-2899

http://www.theclinics.com

PHYSICAL MEDICINE AND REHABILITATION CLINICS OF NORTH AMERICA Volume 26, Number 3
August 2015 ISSN 1047-9651, ISBN 978-0-323-39352-2

Editor: Jennifer Flynn-Briggs
Developmental Editor: Donald Mumford

Reprints. For copies of 100 or more of articles in this publication, please contact the Commercial Reprints Department, Elsevier Inc., 360 Park Avenue South, New York, NY 10010-1710. Tel.: 212-633-3874; Fax: 212-633-3820; E-mail: reprints@elsevier.com.

Physical Medicine and Rehabilitation Clinics of North America (ISSN 1047-9651) is published quarterly by Elsevier Inc., 360 Park Avenue South, New York, NY 10010-1710. Months of issue are February, May, August, and November. Business and Editorial Offices: 1600 John F. Kennedy Blvd., Suite 1800, Philadelphia, PA 19103-2899. Customer Service Office: 3251 Riverport Lane, Maryland Heights, MO 63043. Periodicals postage paid at New York, NY and additional mailing offices. Subscription price per year is $275.00 (US individuals), $486.00 (US institutions), $145.00 (US students), $335.00 (Canadian individuals), $640.00 (Canadian institutions), $210.00 (Canadian students), $415.00 (foreign individuals), $640.00 (foreign institutions), and $210.00 (foreign students). Foreign air speed delivery is included in all *Clinics* subscription prices. All prices are subject to change without notice. **POSTMASTER:** Send address changes to *Physical Medicine and Rehabilitation Clinics of North America*, Customer Service Office: Elsevier Health Sciences Division, Subscription Customer Service, 3251 Riverport Lane, Maryland Heights, MO 63043. **Customer Service: 1-800-654-2452 (US). From outside of the United States, call 314-447-8871. Fax: 314-447-8029. E-mail: JournalsCustomer Service-usa@elsevier.com (for print support); JournalsOnlineSupport-usa@elsevier.com (for online support).**

Physical Medicine and Rehabilitation Clinics of North America is indexed in *Excerpta Medica, MEDLINE/ PubMed (Index Medicus), Cinahl,* and *Cumulative Index to Nursing and Allied Health Literature.*

Contributors

CONSULTING EDITOR

GREGORY T. CARTER, MD, MS
Consulting Medical Editor, Medical Director, St Luke's Rehabilitation Institute, Spokane, Washington; University of Washington, School of Medicine, Seattle, Washington

EDITORS

ANDREW S. FRIEDMAN, MD
Section Head; Clinical Assistant Professor, Departments of Physical Medicine and Rehabilitation and Neuroscience Institute, University of Washington; Virginia Mason Medical Center, Seattle, Washington

GARY M. FRANKLIN, MD, MPH
Medical Director, Washington State Department of Labor and Industries; Research Professor, Departments of Environmental and Occupational Health Sciences, Neurology and Health Services, University of Washington, Seattle, Washington

AUTHORS

CHRISTOPHER H. ALLAN, MD
Associate Professor, Department of Orthopedic Surgery, Hand and Microsurgery Section, Harborview Medical Center, The University of Washington School of Medicine, Seattle, Washington

MICHAEL CODSI, MD
EvergreeenHealth Medical Center, Kirkland, Washington

TERESA COOPER, MN, MPH
Department of Labor and Industries, Olympia, Washington

NIKKI D'URSO, RN
Occupational Nurse Consultant Supervisor; Washington State Department of Labor and Industries, Olympia, Washington

GARY M. FRANKLIN, MD, MPH
Medical Director, Washington State Department of Labor and Industries; Research Professor, Departments of Environmental and Occupational Health Sciences, Neurology and Health Services, University of Washington, Seattle, Washington

ANDREW S. FRIEDMAN, MD
Section Head; Clinical Assistant Professor, Departments of Physical Medicine and Rehabilitation and Neuroscience Institute, University of Washington; Virginia Mason Medical Center, Seattle, Washington

CHRIS R. HOWE, MD
Proliance Orthopedic Associates, Renton, Washington

SIMONE P. JAVAHER, RN, BSN, MPA
Health Policy Clinical Manager, Office of the Medical Director, Labor and Industries, Olympia, Washington

JEAN-CHRISTOPHE A. LEVEQUE, MD
Group Health, Seattle, Washington

JAYMIE MAI, PharmD
Pharmacy Manager, Washington State Department of Labor and Industries, Olympia, Washington

BINTU MARONG-CEESAY, MS
Department of Health, Olympia, Washington

NICHOLAS K. REUL, MD, MPH
Clinical Instructor of Medicine, Department of Occupational and Environmental Medicine, University of Washington; Associate Medical Director for Occupational Disease, Washington State Department of Labor and Industries, Seattle, Washington

LARRY ROBINSON, MD
Chief, Rehabilitation Services; John and Sally Eaton Chair in Rehabilitation Science; Professor, Division Director, Physical Medicine and Rehabilitation, Sunnybrook Health Sciences Centre, University of Toronto, Toronto, Ontario, Canada

HAL STOCKBRIDGE, MD, MPH
Associate Medical Director, Washington State Department of Labor and Industries, Olympia; Clinical Assistant Professor, University of Washington, Seattle, Washington

DAVID TAUBEN, MD
Chief, Division of Pain Medicine; Clinical Associate Professor, Anesthesia and Pain Medicine, University of Washington Medical Center, University of Washington, Seattle, Washington

MICHAEL D. WEISS, MD
Chief, Neuromuscular Division; Professor, Department of Neurology, University of Washington School of Medicine, Seattle, Washington

Contents

> Washington state's public workers' compensation system has had a
> formal process for developing and implementing evidence-based clinical
> practice guidelines since 2007. Collaborating with the Industrial Insurance
> Medical Advisory Committee and clinicians from the medical community,
> the Office of the Medical Director has provided leadership and staff sup-
> port necessary to develop guidelines that have improved outcomes and
> reduced the number of potentially harmful procedures. Guidelines are
> selected according to a prioritization schema and follow a development
> process consistent with that of the national Institute of Medicine. Evalua-
> tion criteria are also applied. Guidelines continue to be developed to
> provide clinical recommendations for optimizing care and reducing risk
> of harm.

> Peer-reviewed medical literature plays a decisive role in policy develop-
> ment at the Washington State Department of Labor and Industries (L&I).
> L&I relies on multiple evidence-based mechanisms to make coverage
> decisions and translate medical science into public policy, including stat-
> ute, rule writing, executive policy, real-time evidence assessment, pilot
> testing, and collaboration with researchers. Elements of L&I's policy pro-
> cess structure and evidence-based culture are also observed in original
> literature discussing the needs and barriers of incorporating evidence
> into public policy.

> The value of treatment guidelines in improving outcomes for patients and
> controlling costs is significantly enhanced in Washington by incorporating
> guidelines into a structured UR program. This article describes: (1) how the

diminished sensation or dysesthesias in the fourth or fifth digits, often coupled with pain in the proximal medial aspect of the elbow. Treatment may be conservative or surgical, but optimal management remains controversial. Surgery should include exploration of the ulnar nerve throughout its course around the elbow and release of all compressive structures.

Carpal tunnel syndrome is the most common entrapment neuropathy, and its risk of occurrence in the presence of repetitive, forceful angular hand movements, or vibration, is common. It is critical to make the diagnosis based on appropriate clinical history and findings and with corroborating electrodiagnostic studies. Conservative management should be undertaken with the goal of maintaining employment; surgical decompression can be highly effective, particularly if undertaken early on.

Proximal median (PMNE) and radial (RNE) nerve entrapment syndromes are uncommon. This article provides an evidenced-based treatment guideline for PMNE and RNE based on the available literature. Arriving at an accurate diagnosis must involve an electrodiagnostic (EDx) workup. EDx, including nerve conduction velocity studies and needle electromyography, should corroborate the clinical diagnosis and must be done before consideration of any surgical treatment. Conservative care includes rest, modified activities, splinting at wrist and elbow, physical therapy, antiinflammatory drug therapy, and corticosteroid injections. Conservative care should be required for at least 6 weeks before any operative interventions are considered.

Outcomes of surgery for neurogenic thoracic outlet syndrome (NTOS) in workers' compensation are poor in a majority of patients, partly due to nonspecificity of diagnosis. Most cases have no objective evidence of the presence of brachial plexus dysfunction. Up to 20% of patients experience a new adverse event. Objective neurologic signs and electrodiagnostic evidence of brachial plexus dysfunction must be present before proceeding with invasive procedures. This guideline includes objective criteria that must be met before thoracic outlet syndrome surgery can be approved in Washington State. Evidence does not support the use of scalene blocks, botulinum toxin therapy, or vascular studies to diagnose NTOS.

Complex regional pain syndrome can be a debilitating disorder, which, in its earliest stages, can be prevented by aggressive rehabilitation based on reactivation. It is critical to follow international criteria on making the diagnosis; overdiagnosis can lead to inappropriate interventions and further disability. When present, early recognition with reactivation is the cornerstone of treatment. This article presents a phased approach to treatment that suggests movements of nonresponders quickly to more integrated levels of care. Some commonly used invasive interventions, such as sympathectomy and spinal cord stimulation, have not been proved effective; these unproven and potentially harmful therapies should be avoided.

PHYSICAL MEDICINE AND REHABILITATION CLINICS OF NORTH AMERICA

VISIT THE CLINICS ONLINE!
Access your subscription at:
www.theclinics.com

Foreword

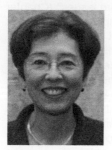

Dianna Chamblin, MD

There are more medical treatment guidelines than Carter's proverbial pills (no relation to our illustrious editor). In the National Guideline Clearinghouse (NGC) alone, there are several thousand guidelines. What sets guidelines apart to add value and utility to the busy provider? The Washington State Workers' Compensation System (Department of Labor and Industries or L&I) appears to have found the recipe for success by focusing on collaboration, consensus, and transparency throughout the development process. Their "secret sauce" is a process that allows all users a voice in development, well before implementation. The evaluation and treatment recommendations in these guidelines are applicable to both occupational and nonoccupational-related conditions.

L&I is one of many Washington State public agencies, but is the only insurer for its citizens when they incur illnesses or injuries in the course of working for Washington-based employers. Employers may choose to self-insure their claims, but all state employers must adhere to the same state statutes and agency regulations. Guideline topics are prioritized based on several criteria, such as patient safety concerns, treatment outcomes, variations in practice quality, and business needs, such as consistency with other state or federal decisions, or simply the need to update them due to new compelling medical evidence or NGC expiration dates.

L&I first developed treatment guidelines in 1989 with assistance from the Washington State Medical Association. The first guideline established admission criteria for the inpatient treatment of nonsurgical back pain. Within one year, these admissions fell by 60%. Twenty-five years later, it is even difficult to remember or conceive of the time when patients with acute lumbar radiculopathies were hospitalized for bed rest, traction, and analgesics.

Over the years, L&I guidelines have further evolved into a highly collaborative and more formalized process by inviting input and direction from the Industrial Insurance Medical Advisory Committee (IIMAC). IIMAC was established by the legislature and formed in 2007. The statute empowers IIMAC to: "Advise the department on matters related to the provision of safe, effective, and cost-effective treatments for injured

Phys Med Rehabil Clin N Am 26 (2015) xi–xiii
http://dx.doi.org/10.1016/j.pmr.2015.05.002
1047-9651/15/$ – see front matter © 2015 Published by Elsevier Inc.

workers, including but not limited to the development of practice guidelines and coverage criteria, review of coverage decisions and technology assessments, review of medical programs and review of rules pertaining to health care issues" (Chapter 51.36 RCW). Comprised of practicing clinicians from varied specialties who are educated about evidence-based medicine, IIMAC members meet with L&I representatives quarterly in a forum open to the public. A clinical epidemiologist extensively combs for relevant, peer-reviewed medical literature and categorizes the articles using the American Academy of Neurology grading criteria. IIMAC members, additional subject matter experts, researchers, and policymakers join together as a subcommittee and sift through the literature to create the initial guideline drafts. The guideline drafts are reviewed by the parent IIMAC, and by the most critical reviewers: the general public. The comments received are addressed until the final guideline product is approved and posted on the L&I website: www.lni.wa.gov. Further details of this process are described in the article written by Simone Javaher, BSN, MPA, Health Policy Clinical Manager at L&I.

Guideline implementation has resulted in clearer definitions of evidenced-based care and reduction of unnecessary surgeries, diagnostic testing, and treatment. For example, there has been a 74% reduction in proximal median nerve entrapment release surgeries three years after implementation of the proximal median nerve entrapment guideline; a 48% reduction in thoracic outlet surgeries four years after the effective date of thoracic outlet syndrome guideline; and a 67% reduction in radial tunnel surgeries three years after implementation of the radial tunnel guideline. Although reduction of surgery alone is not the desired objective of the guidelines, reduction of surgery in the absence of objective evidence-based criteria that improve outcomes and reduce harm for patients is the intent. Risk of harm is defined as a pattern of low-quality care that exposes patients to the risk of physical or psychiatric harm or death.

Transparency of the guideline processes and definitions of best practice treatments have additionally complemented L&I's other successful efforts in disability prevention programs, such as the establishment of Centers for Occupational Health and Education (COHEs). This innovative effort is aimed directly at improving quality of care delivered via incenting occupational best practices and dedicated health services coordination. The combination of using best evidence and a consensus of expert opinion to produce guidelines and coverage decisions and health care innovation via the COHEs is highly likely to help reduce the chance of a worker losing his or her life to disability from routine musculoskeletal injuries.

As Chair of the IIMAC, past Chair of various guideline subcommittees, Medical Director of the Everett COHE, and a practicing clinician, the adoption of inclusive, transparent, and collaborative approaches to improve patient care with an insurer has been a welcomed partnership. Together, we are able to use the best available medical evidence and needs of the injured worker as our compass in producing guidelines that meet the rigors of multiple reviewers from many perspectives. The reduction of inappropriate, ineffective, or further disabling care has been a welcomed by-product for all who hold the patient's best interest at heart.

May you find value and guidance in this collection of very high-level evidence-based guidelines, created and supported by national experts and assembled by L&I's Medical Director, Dr Gary Franklin, and IIMAC Vice Chair, Dr Andrew Friedman, guest editors of this issue of the *Physical Medicine and Rehabilitation Clinics of North America.*

Dianna Chamblin, MD
The Everett Clinic Occupational Medicine Department
Center for Occupational Health
and Education at The Everett Clinic
Industrial Insurance Medical Advisory Committee
The Everett Clinic
4027 Hoyt Avenue, Suite 104
Everett, WA 98201, USA

E-mail address:
dchamblin@everettclinic.com

Editorial

Evidence-Based Guidelines in Workers' Compensation

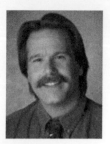

Gregory T. Carter, MD, MS
Consulting Editor

I want to extend my sincerest thanks to the editors of this issue of *Physical Medicine and Rehabilitation Clinics of North America*, Drs Andrew Friedman and Gary Franklin. I also want to thank all of the authors who contributed to this very special issue. Under the progressive, forward-thinking leadership of Dr Franklin and his team at the Department of Labor and Industries, the Industrial Insurance Medical Advisory Committee (IIMAC) was formed in 2007. The Washington State Legislature authorizes the IIMAC to advise the Department of Labor and Industries on matters related to the provision of safe, effective, and cost-effective treatments for injured workers, including but not limited to the development of practice guidelines and coverage criteria, review of coverage decisions and technology assessments, review of medical programs, and review of rules pertaining to health care issues. This issue represents some of the best work from the IIMAC, and I think clinicians will find this text remarkably useful.

Gregory T. Carter, MD, MS
St Luke's Rehabilitation Institute
711 South Cowley Street
Spokane, WA 99202, USA

E-mail address:
gtcarter@uw.edu

Note from the Publisher: On behalf of Elsevier and Physical Medicine and Rehabilitation Clinics, I would like to thank Dr. Carter for his years of service, dedication, and contributions to the publication. The August 2015 issue of Physical Medicine and Rehabilitation Clinics will be the last one under Dr. Carter's editorship. We would like to wish him well in all his future endeavors.
  Jennifer Flynn-Briggs,
  Senior Clinics Editor, Physical Medicine and Rehabilitation Clinics

Phys Med Rehabil Clin N Am 26 (2015) xv
http://dx.doi.org/10.1016/j.pmr.2015.05.003
1047-9651/15/$ – see front matter © 2015 Published by Elsevier Inc.

pmr.theclinics.com

Preface

Evidence-based Guidelines in Workers' Compensation

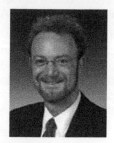   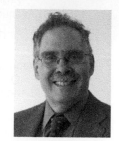

Andrew S. Friedman, MD   Gary M. Franklin, MD, MPH
Editors

This issue was developed as a means to disseminate what we believe to be the highest quality guidelines available for common and controversial conditions in workers' compensation. Many, of course, can be applied more generally in treating conditions outside of the injured worker population.

While scientific evidence is dramatically increasing, it is rarely adequate to address the complex and variable issues surrounding even the most common medical conditions and injuries. This makes the development of guidelines to address those conditions both challenging and critically important. Although it is often difficult to incorporate guidelines into medical management decisions and payment policies, that is the exact goal of these Washington State efforts. Importantly, providers and patients recognize that individual patient circumstances may significantly impact how a general guideline is applied, so great consideration is given to this in their writing and application.

This issue describes not only the specific guideline recommendations for common medical conditions in workers' compensation but also the methods and processes used to develop them. The collaboration among state government leaders, medical advisors, community physicians and clinicians, and utilization review teams is an exemplary model of cooperation that ensures the guidelines are clear and clinically relevant. After vetting them with the public and after approval by Labor and Industries' statutory Industrial Insurance Medical Advisory Committee in an open public meeting, these guidelines are in the public domain and available to all. (Labor and Industries is the department that administers Washington State's workers' compensation system.)

Phys Med Rehabil Clin N Am 26 (2015) xvii–xviii
http://dx.doi.org/10.1016/j.pmr.2015.05.001
1047-9651/15/$ – see front matter © 2015 Published by Elsevier Inc.

This approach enables those who use them to make sound clinical decisions from a blend of the best medical evidence and expert opinion so that ultimately the best care reaches the worker.

We sincerely hope you find this issue useful.

Andrew S. Friedman, MD
Virginia Mason Medical Center
1100 9th Avenue, Seattle, WA 98111, USA

Gary M. Franklin, MD, MPH
University of Washington
Department of Environmental and
Occupational Health Sciences
130 Nickerson Street, Suite 212
Seattle, WA 98109, USA

E-mail addresses:
Andrew.friedman@virginiamason.org (A.S. Friedman)
meddir@uw.edu (G.M. Franklin)

Guideline Development Process in a Public Workers' Compensation System

Simone P. Javaher, RN, BSN, MPA

KEYWORDS

- Medical guideline • Treatment guideline • Clinical practice guideline
- Workers' compensation • Injured workers

KEY POINTS

- Evidence-based clinical practice guidelines are developed and implemented in Washington state workers' compensation using a rigorous and transparent process.
- Collaboration, dedicated staff, transparency, and process integrity are keys to success.
- Community clinicians partner with government in the development of these guidelines, leading to their broad acceptance.

INTRODUCTION

Evidence-based medicine has become the generally accepted approach in today's health care system for determining what constitutes safe, effective, and cost-effective care, whereas in the past, it was more likely to be "eminence-based medicine" (ie, relying on opinions from senior clinicians without any standardized process and safeguards against bias).[1–3] The caveat with evidence-based medicine is that the advent of new technologies, devices, surgical techniques, and emerging or alternative treatments outpaces the availability of high-quality unbiased research such that it is often insufficient to support the use of these health services. Formally developed clinical practice guidelines help fill this gap, although even rigorously developed guidelines do not ensure they will be accepted in clinical practice.[4] Since 1992, when the national Institute of Medicine (IOM) published its report, "Guidelines for Clinical Practice: From Development to Use," the number of evidence-based clinical practice guidelines has skyrocketed. The Guidelines International Network (GIN) was founded in 2002 and has since counted (6509 guidelines across 96 organizations in 79

Conflicts of Interest: None.
Office of the Medical Director, Labor and Industries, PO Box 44321, Olympia, WA 98504-4321, USA
E-mail address: Simone.javaher@Lni.wa.gov

Phys Med Rehabil Clin N Am 26 (2015) 427–434
http://dx.doi.org/10.1016/j.pmr.2015.04.009
1047-9651/15/$ – see front matter © 2015 Elsevier Inc. All rights reserved.

pmr.theclinics.com

countries as of May 2015[5]). The challenge is translating the plethora of scientific evidence into recommendations that are useful for the everyday practitioner.

The National Guideline Clearinghouse (NGC), which is part of the US Health and Human Services Agency for Healthcare Research and Quality, maintains a central repository of national and international guidelines based on inclusion criteria established by the IOM in 2008.[6] **Fig. 1** illustrates this trend.

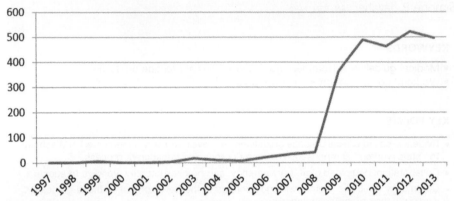

Fig. 1. Number of new guidelines published each year on the NGC. (*Data from* Javaher SP. National Guideline Clearinghouse. Available at: www.guideline.gov. Accessed December 13, 2014.)

These guidelines are not a substitute for sound clinical decision making; rather, they inform and facilitate sound clinical decision making. If developed using a rigorous method, clinical practice guidelines can provide easy-to-follow criteria, algorithms, and decision-making tools that help optimize patient care, improve treatment outcomes, and prevent harm. Although they are based on scientific evidence, they also draw on the expertise of researchers, clinicians, policy makers, and myriad others who can dive deeply into critical questions and nuances that the literature may not elucidate. Although variation exists among expert opinions and experience, systematically synthesized information derived from high-quality studies and a consensus of expert opinion can enhance the individual provider's ability to deliver high-quality care. In addition, by using a transparent, rigorous, and trustworthy process, guidelines can have greater relevance and credibility for the clinician and withstand scrutiny in the era of accountable care.

Since the 1980s, the Office of the Medical Director (OMD) in Washington state's workers' compensation system (part of Department of Labor and Industries [L&I]) has developed clinical practice guidelines (called medical treatment guidelines [MTGs]), and was the first workers' compensation program to publish them on the NGC in 2002. To date, Colorado is the only other public workers' compensation agency to post their guidelines on the NGC (starting in 2009). OMDs guidelines are used in the utilization review (UR) program and are regularly reviewed and updated as necessary. Furthermore, providers who treat Washington's injured workers must be in our network and as such, are required by statute to use our MTGs (Revised Code of Washington 51.36.010). This article describes the rigorous guideline development process that OMD has refined during the last 7 years, which grew out of a model of collaboration and cooperation with our medical advisors, the health care community, and the public. These partnerships have been rewarding and crucial to the success of our work.

HOW IT STARTED

In 2007, the Industrial Insurance Medical Advisory Committee (IIMAC) was formed through passage of agency-sponsored legislation (SSB 5801, CH 6 [2011]; codified as Revised Code of Washington 51.36.140). Fourteen physicians are nominated by their specialty societies or institutions and appointed by the L&I director to be members. These physicians are required to be practicing clinicians representing family medicine, orthopedics, neurology, neurosurgery, general surgery, physical medicine and rehabilitation, psychiatry, internal medicine, osteopathic, pain medicine, and occupational medicine. At least two are required to have special expertise in evidence-based medicine. Although such a committee could have been formed by agency executive action, the statute provided two unique legal authorities: members are protected from legal action by the full extent of State legal authority; and members may be reimbursed for their work. In addition, all IIMAC meetings must be open to the public, so transparency is a built-in expectation.

The law also established an Industrial Insurance Chiropractic Advisory Committee (IICAC), charged with using evidence to ensure workers receive high-quality chiropractic care. IICAC members are also nominated from their professional societies and institutions, and they follow a similar rigorous process for developing conservative care "practice resources" that summarize available evidence for common occupational musculoskeletal conditions. These practice resources complement the IIMAC guidelines and are also included on the NGC Web site (www.guidelines. gov).

Led by an IIMAC member with expertise in the chosen topic, specially assigned subcommittees are formed to develop MTGs. Additional clinicians who are highly recognized leaders in the community are invited to complement subcommittee's expertise. All clinical contributors to the guidelines must not have financial or nonfinancial conflicts of interest, and outside sponsorship or funding of a guideline is never accepted. The effectiveness and popularity of the IIMAC and IICAC work have generated so much interest that there is a waiting list of providers who want to join them. The success of OMD is largely because of agency leadership that led to the statutory establishment of these partnerships with community providers, dedicated resources to build staff capacity, and integrity in the guideline development process. But the glue that binds these elements together to truly make it work is constructive engagement, trust, and high-quality work, making the highest level of collaboration possible (**Box 1**). In February 2015, the IIMAC began work on its 15th guideline.

Box 1
Hallmarks of success

1. Leadership/statutory authority

2. Dedicated resources

3. Collaboration

4. Transparency

5. Process integrity

SELECTION CRITERIA

Guideline development begins with prioritizing and selecting the topics. In consultation with IIMAC advisors and the L&I UR program managers and vendor, prioritization is based on the following criteria:

- Is there a cause for concern?
  a. Patient safety: is there a quality concern that poses a risk to the patient?
  b. Efficacy: are we seeing poor outcome data?
  c. Utilization and cost: what is the prevalence?
  d. Practice variation: is there wide variation from best practice?
  e. Rapidly emerging or diffusing technology: what are the implications?
- What are the business needs?
  a. From our partners: IIMAC members, clinicians, or self-insured employers?
  b. In our UR program?
  c. Controversy regarding a procedure, technology, or device?
  d. Legal requirements (eg, decisions or rulings from state and federal agencies)?
- Can we leverage resources?
  a. Can we group guidelines that require the same medical specialists?
  b. Are other state agencies and payers working on an issue/guideline for which there may be a mutual interest?
- How old is the guideline?
  a. Does new scientific literature indicate an update is needed? Has there been a sudden increase in cost and utilization, or is it due to expire on the NGC (must be updated every 5 years)?

The typical view of an insurer's role in using guidelines is that they are intended to save money. Although cost and use patterns may be a factor in selecting what guideline to develop, they are rarely primary influences. The mission of OMD is to help injured workers heal and return to work by ensuring appropriate high-quality care is provided and harm is avoided. To preserve the integrity of these goals, OMD is separated from that part of the agency that regulates reimbursement for health care services. Furthermore, Washington has many statewide evidence-based health care policy and purchasing requirements so there are built-in checks and balances for accuracy, consistency, and quality. Additionally, the workers' compensation program has a long-standing research relationship with the University of Washington's Occupational and Environmental Health Program to independently investigate, evaluate, and inform many of the agency's guideline development efforts. This has established an iterative culture of policy needs informing research agendas and research findings informing policy development. Most importantly, this unique capacity to inform guideline development with outcomes research has led to improved outcomes for injured workers.[7]

DEVELOPMENT PROCESS

There are two ways to discuss this process: the standards we use, and how we go about implementing them. We follow most of the standards set by the IOM for developing trustworthy clinical practice guidelines (**Box 2**).

Once a guideline topic is selected and the scope and objectives are identified, we begin the process of actual development. First, our epidemiologist does a systematic review of the literature based on key words and questions, and summarizes the findings into evidence tables using the grading schema from the American Academy of Neurology.[8] Then, over the course of 3 to 5 months, the epidemiologist and OMD

Box 2
Institute of Medicine's guideline development standards

1. Establish transparency
2. Management and disclosure of conflict of interest
3. Multidisciplinary and diverse group participation
4. Systematic review of the literature
5. Strength rating for the clinical recommendations
6. Clearly articulated clinical recommendations
7. External review of guidelines
8. Keeping guidelines updated

Data from Institute of Medicine. Clinical practice guidelines we can trust. In: Graham R, et al, editors. Washington, DC: The National Academies Press; 2011. p. 33–4.

---

clinical staff meet with IIMAC subcommittee members, invited consulting practitioners, and clinicians from our UR vendor to hammer out the language and criteria. Each guideline typically includes the sections shown in **Box 3**, some of which are customized for an injured worker population.

Box 3
Typical table of contents in Washington state's workers' compensation guideline

A. Introduction
B. Establishing work-relatedness
C. Making the diagnosis
   1. Case definition (symptoms and signs)
   2. Relevant diagnostic tests (eg, imaging, electrodiagnostic, laboratory, and so forth)
D. Clinical recommendations
   1. Conservative treatment
   2. Surgical treatment
E. Return to work
   1. Early assessment, including occupational health quality indicators
   2. Returning to work following surgery
F. Worksheets, tools, forms
G. Guideline summary or algorithm for professional nurse reviewers (this may be at the start)

Subcommittee members critique and revise the draft guideline language as it is developed based on what is most useful for the clinician, the UR program, and any additional evidence or expert opinions that are brought to their attention. This typically means creating evaluation and review criteria in a table format so the recommendations are clear and easy to use. A final draft of the guideline is posted on the agency Web site for public comment for 4 weeks. After all public comments are received and reviewed, responses are provided by the subcommittee and posted on the Web site.

The subcommittee may make further revisions to the draft guideline until they present the final draft to the full advisory committee during one of its quarterly public meetings. Any member of the public can give oral comments at the meeting and changes may still be made. Once the full committee makes the advisory recommendation to adopt the guideline, OMD makes the final decision, and it usually becomes final 30 days later.

Although we do not typically involve injured workers in the development process, they can access and comment on the guidelines when they are posted online or presented at the full IIMAC meeting. It is more our statutory relationships with business and labor leaders that give the process a great deal of credibility in our workers' compensation authorizing environment.

Strength ratings of published scientific evidence are typically included; however, our process does not try to summarize overall strength of recommendations. This is rather unique to a public process of guideline development where the expectation is that guidelines serve as provider education and as review criteria for our UR vendor.[5] The latter requires specific enough guidance to allow a coverage decision to be made; highly nuanced summaries of strength of recommendations would make such decisions in the public sector very difficult.

Every guideline has limitations, and a guideline that is too technical or overly comprehensive can create a burden when clinicians try to adopt it, leading to underuse of otherwise excellent evidence-based guidance. Thus, in addition to internal and external validity, including expert consensus by respected community clinicians gives face validity to the guideline, resulting in clear recommendations that are user-friendly and acceptable to the clinician.

IMPLEMENTATION AND UPDATES

Probably equal to the challenge of writing guidelines, is making sure there is implementation validity in that they can be put into practice at all levels (eg, in the clinic, by the UR vendor, and by claim adjudicators). At L&I, most guidelines are implemented within the UR program. Although proprietary guidelines and criteria may be used, L&I guidelines have priority because they are highly credible within our health care provider community. Reviewers apply each guideline as a standard for most requests.

Effective communication is also an integral part of the implementation process. The communication plan includes health care providers, claim managers, our UR staff and vendor, policy makers within the agency, and our self-insured employers and their third-party administrators (which account for about a third of Washington's workforce). We share guidelines at conferences and CME courses, and we post them on the L&I external Web site, which in 2014 had 85,441 downloads (70,315 medical and 15,126 chiropractic) on the L&I Web site alone (www.lni.wa.gov).

With the ongoing changes in health technologies and procedures and emerging scientific evidence, and with the continued need to devote resources to new guidelines, we keep to a schedule of regular review of the guidelines as they age. We depend heavily on our epidemiologist for this review and revision work, and all potential changes and updates are presented to the full IIMAC for their recommendations.

GUIDELINE EVALUATION

Evaluating the quality and impact of our guidelines is also part of our process. We informally follow evaluation criteria, such as that provided by Appraisal of Guidelines for Research and Evaluation II, which is fairly straightforward because it is complimentary to the IOM process criteria (**Box 4**)

Box 4
Six domains of Appraisal of Guidelines for Research and Evaluation II evaluation criteria

1. Explicit scope and purpose (clear objective and clear target population)

2. Stakeholder involvement (Appraisal of Guidelines for Research and Evaluation II also cites patient involvement, but we use provider involvement)

3. Rigor of development (proper use of evidence, external review, guards against bias, risks vs benefits are considered)

4. Clarity of presentation (clinical recommendations are easy to identify and use, summary tables, and so forth)

5. Applicability (impacts, costs, and monitoring)

6. Editorial independence (no industry funding or conflicts of interest among developers)

Data from Institute of Medicine. Clinical practice guidelines we can trust. In: Graham R, et al, editors. Washington, DC: The National Academies Press; 2011. p. 33–4.

Evaluating the impact of our guidelines on the quality of care received by injured workers is complex. We know that surgical guidelines work when approved requests for workers who truly require surgery increase, and requests are denied when the worker's clinical presentation does not meet the guideline's criteria. Additionally, we know our guidelines provide educational value to providers around the world. In the future, we may offer financial incentives for providers to use our guidelines as a measure of occupational medicine best practices. We continue to look for ways to evaluate their impact on more hard to get-at data, such as how readily correct diagnoses are made, or the extent to which disability is reduced, or whether they help prevent overuse of opioids. As technology changes (eg, the adoption of electronic medical records and the availability of prescription monitoring programs) it is possible we can gain these insights in the future, so Washington's workers' compensation program will continue to resource this important and effective effort. Visit the L&I Web site to review our guidelines and our IIMAC committee work at www.lni. wa.gov.

SUMMARY/DISCUSSION

Whether they are called clinical practice or medical treatment guidelines, and whether they are developed by a government agency, a for-profit organization, or a private nonprofit professional association, the common goal is to produce "recommendations intended to optimize patient care that are informed by a systematic review of evidence and an assessment of the benefits and harms of alternative care options."[1] Although motives and methods may vary, guideline authors must stay true to the principles of evidence-based medicine and quality guideline standards so practitioners who make the day-to-day clinical decisions have current, valid, and reliable information. The days of "eminence-based medicine" are gone, and guideline developers cannot properly evaluate the benefits of a guideline unless clinicians adopt and apply them. Guidelines need to have an institutional home where a process of developing trustworthy guidelines can be sustained.[2] In Washington, the workers' compensation system has established this institutional home in the L&I OMD. Through collaboration with a statutory advisory committee, dedicated resources, collaboration, transparency, and process integrity, a successful method of producing high-quality MTGs has been established and its future for continued improvement is ensured.

REFERENCES

1. Institute of Medicine. Clinical practice guidelines we can trust. In: Graham R, Mancher M, Wolman DM, et al, editors. Washington, DC: The National Academies Press; 2011. p. 33–4.
2. Ransohoff DF, Pignone M, Sox HC. How to decide whether a clinical practice guideline is worthy. JAMA 2013;309:139–40.
3. Szajewska H. Clinical practice guidelines: based on eminence or evidence? Ann Nutr Metab 2014;64:325–31.
4. Nuckols TK, Yee-Wei L, Wynn BO. Rigorous development does not ensure that guidelines are acceptable to a panel of knowledgeable providers. J Gen Intern Med 2007;23:37–44.
5. Guidelines International Network. Resources/international guideline library. guidelines international network. 2011. Available at: http://www.g-i-n.net/library/international-guidelines-library. Accessed December 13, 2014.
6. Institute of Medicine. Committee on reviewing evidence to identify highly effective clinical services. In: Eden J, Wheatley B, McNeil B, et al, editors. Knowing what works in health care, a roadmap for the nation. Washington, DC: The National Academies Press; 2008. Available at: http://www.guideline.gov/about/inclusion-criteria.aspx. Accessed May 15, 2015.
7. Martin BI, Franklin GM, Deyo RA. How do coverage policies influence practice patterns, safety, and cost of initial lumbar fusion surgery? A population-based comparison of workers' compensation systems. Spine J 2014;14:1237–46.
8. American Academy of Neurology. Clinical practice guideline process manual. St Paul (MN): The American Academy of Neurology; 2011.

Introduction to Evidence-Based Decision Making in a Public Workers' Compensation Agency

CrossMark

Nicholas K. Reul, MD, MPH[a,b,*]

KEYWORDS

- Evidence based • Public policy • Workers' compensation • Policy development
- Industrial insurance

KEY POINTS

- Successful policy development and implementation are associated with needs distinct from those of individual clinical encounters.
- The principles of evidence-based medicine remain valuable when applied to population health concerns.
- Characteristics of Washington's Department of Labor and Industries (L&I) promote the inclusion of original research and evidence-based medicine principles that contribute to quality policy development.
- Washington relies on evidence-based policy to direct resources toward those interventions that work.

INTRODUCTION

The Department of Labor and Industries (L&I) is charged with allocating industrial insurance resources to deliver "sure and certain relief for workers, injured in their work, and their families and dependents."[1] To ensure the responsible stewardship of these resources on behalf of the public, L&I uses as a guide the principle that resources should be directed toward those interventions that work, redirecting resources away from ineffective practices. The paradigm shift and tools that have accompanied the ascendance of the evidence-based medicine movement lend natural support to this objective, consistent with the movement's goals of deemphasizing "intuition, unsystematic clinical experience, and pathophysiologic rationale as

a Department of Occupational and Environmental Medicine, University of Washington, Box 359739, 325 9th Avenue, Seattle, WA 98104, USA; b Washington State Department of Labor and Industries, Office of the Medical Director, PO Box 44315, Olympia, WA 98504-4315, USA
* Department of Occupational and Environmental Medicine, University of Washington, Box 359739, 325 9th Avenue, Seattle, WA 98104, USA.
E-mail address: nreul@uw.edu

Phys Med Rehabil Clin N Am 26 (2015) 435–443
http://dx.doi.org/10.1016/j.pmr.2015.04.010
1047-9651/15/$ – see front matter © 2015 Elsevier Inc. All rights reserved.

sufficient grounds for clinical decision making" as well as to stress "the examination of evidence from clinical research."[2]

Defined as "the conscientious, explicit and judicious use of current best evidence in making decisions about the care of individual patients, [t]he practice of evidence-based medicine means integrating individual clinical expertise with the best available external clinical evidence from systematic research."[3] To reap the benefits of the research that is the underpinning of evidence-based medicine, L&I has formalized the use of evidence throughout the methods the agency uses to translate medical research into the public policies that protect injured workers and prevent the development and progression of disability.

As a public health agency, regulator, and implementer of policies targeting the health of the entire injured worker population in Washington State, the scope of L&I's work is necessarily population based, and is thus broader than the integration of clinical acumen and external systematic research on behalf of individual patients described by Sackett and colleagues.[3] Such a population perspective brings with it peculiar needs, the consideration of which continue to be articulated in recent literature recommending the principles and actions that evidence-based medicine should incorporate to best serve patients.[4]

The evidence-based policy literature describes multiple barriers perceived to impair the successful use of academic research in policy development for public health entities, such as L&I. After describing some of those barriers, this article details several of the organizational characteristics and process solutions that have permitted the agency to overcome such hurdles, giving rise to the decisive role that peer-reviewed medical literature now plays in policy development at L&I.

PUBLIC POLICY AND THE TRANSLATION OF EVIDENCE

Translating the research foundation on which evidence-based medicine rests into public health policy entails difficulties. As Rütten[5] explains, "there are several papers emphasizing that the 'golden standard' of evidence-based medicine, with a certain hierarchy of evidence and an emphasis on randomized control trials (RCTs), does not fit well to evidence-based policy." Distinguishing between the effectiveness of policies containing interventions deemed effective from the effectiveness of those interventions, Rütten[5] also concludes "that interventions proven to be most effective at population level will have no chance to affect the population if the respective policy processes fail to implement them properly."[5]

Other investigators have also commented on the broader demands made of evidence-based material by the needs of public policy. Boaz and colleagues[6] note that "reviews are now being undertaken for quite diverse purposes. They do not just seek to answer the 'What works?' questions that have been considered to be appropriate to medicine. In public policy even that question must be reformulated as 'What works, for whom, in what circumstances?'"[6] In addition, in considering guidelines and coverage policies based on available evidence, public agencies must consider 3 dimensions of evidence: effectiveness, harms, and costs, as is the case with the Health Technology Assessment Program described later.

The character of the policy process also figures prominently in such discourse. Incorporating the research base of evidence-based medicine into health policy that successfully brings the benefits of interventions to populations of people invokes additional considerations not necessarily at work in the decisions made by the individual provider and patient. For example, Bartlett[7] describes how "policy-making is not a rational linear process going from the definition of ends, the gathering of evidence, the formulation of a solution and to its implementation. Rather, policy takes place in a context of bounded rationality, in which political decisions are subject to conflicting pressures from advocacy coalitions and policy transfer from external agencies and institutions." Or, as Solesbury[8] explains it, evidence-based policy must answer more than just "what works," but also "what is going on? what's the problem? is it better or worse than...? what causes it? what might be done about it? at what cost? by whose agency?"

Researchers have articulated barriers to successful policy as well as factors that may contribute to success[9–11]:

- Visionary leadership
- Personal relationships/contacts with researchers
- Accessible, clearly presented research
- Policy process transparency
- Structured methods to include and analyze relevant and influential data
- Incentivize change; support with training, technical help
- Use demonstrative pilots
- Provide mechanisms to diffuse the knowledge and skill necessary to produce durable change

FRAMEWORKS OF CHANGE: MEETING THE POLICY NEEDS OF SOCIETY

L&I is not immune to some of the difficulties that come with incorporating original research evidence into establishing public policy.[9,12] The agency's committees (described later) have finite capacities, emphasizing the importance of L&I leadership and its role of prioritizing recommendations for topic selection, thereby furthering its mission and remaining responsive to the needs of the public. Beyond intervention effectiveness, cost and the tradeoffs of resource allocation also figure importantly in implementation planning. Published research is often not designed to answer all the relevant questions that policies need to address, which may dictate choice in policy process: the Health Technology Assessment Program prioritizes topics for which there exists adequate evidence to conduct a complete review.[13] Policy questions may also require a response in less time than a comprehensive review would take.

To address such concerns L&I uses multiple evidence-based processes to deliver coverage policies (**Box 1**), processes that incorporate many characteristics associated with successful evidence-based policy development:

Although coverage policies and guidelines can address most cases, exceptions to policy may arise when clinical circumstances do not neatly fit existing criteria. For these cases, a robust internal review by occupational health nurses and consulting clinicians (eg, Doctor of Medicine, Doctor of Chiropractic, Doctor of Dental Science) helps determine coverage responsibility. In addition to the evidence-based approaches outlined in **Box 1** and these internal review methods, another path may be through the judicial appeals system, wherein a worker or provider may appeal an undesired coverage decision. Although this path ensures reasonable reconsideration for a denied procedure or treatment, the standard is preponderance of evidence based on dueling opinions: the stronger the legal underpinning of evidence-based decisions at the outset, the less likely the need for this judicial process, which is not necessarily as evidence based.

STATUTORY AUTHORITY

Bills passed by the Washington State Legislature and signed into law by the Governor create the statutes that frame Washington's industrial insurance system and provide

---

Box 1
Evidence-based mechanisms for public policy development for health care coverage policy

Statutory authority (eg, Prescription Drug Program, Health Technology Assessment Program, Bree Collaborative)

Agency regulatory authority (eg, definitions of proper and necessary care, including requirements for substantial improvement in pain and function outcomes)

Agency executive policy authority (eg, treatment guidelines, opioid regulations)

Real-time evidence assessment (eg, epidemiologic research on causation, research on emerging issues such as Ebola, research in response to legislative inquiries)

Pilot testing (eg, Centers of Occupational Health and Education [COHEs], occupational health best practices)

L&I-funded research, including at the University of Washington: outcomes research, evaluation research (eg, of COHEs), epidemiologic research, research on risk factors for disability

---

the legal mandate for L&I's work. Consistent with the intent of successive governors and legislatures, L&I's evidence-based approach is substantially authorized in such statutes. **Box 2** summarizes the 5 key evidence-based statutes that authorize all public agencies in Washington State that purchase or regulate health care delivery to implement effective evidence-based coverage policies.

As a state agency, policy development at L&I is supported by the work of all of the statutes in **Box 2**, the most prominent of which are the Prescription Drug Program and the Health Technology Assessment (HTA) program. The Prescription Drug Program has been instrumental in establishing a state formulary for preferred drugs; as a result, L&I now has a 94% generic use rate for drugs. This outcome has led to a total drug expenditure that is 40% less than that experienced across 17 other states workers' compensation programs after adjustment for duration.[14]

The HTA program is charged with evaluating up to 8 health technologies per year with respect to their safety, efficacy, and cost-effectiveness. Decisions the independent health technology clinical committee renders under this program become binding on all Washington State public purchasers of health care. In addition to facilitating unified, evidence-based health policy and coverage decisions by Washington's state agencies, the program is designed to be transparent, to eliminate bias through

---

Box 2
Authority for evidence-based purchasing in Washington State public agencies

2003: Substitute senate bill (SSB) 6088 established the Prescription Drug Program for all agencies; uses evidence within drug classes to determine coverage

2003: Substitute house bill (SHB) 1299; all agencies to conduct formal assessment of scientific evidence to inform coverage, track outcomes, and coordinate efforts

2005: Budget proviso. Agencies to collaborate on coverage and criteria (guidelines); off-label gabapentin done August 2005; opioid dosing guideline, June 2010

2006: Governor request legislation HB 2575/SB 6306 to establish State Health Technology Assessment Program

2011: HB 1311 establishes public/private (Bree) collaborative on guidelines and research, including antitrust protection

independent assessment of evidence, and to rereview existing decisions to remain responsive to evolution in the technologies under evaluation.[15] The statute that provides the framework for the HTA program requires an independent evidence vendor to provide the systematic evaluation of the safety, efficacy, and cost-effectiveness of the technology in question, an additional expense that directly speaks to sensitivity about the importance of systematically presenting primary evidence in an unbiased fashion in support of policy development[7] and provides an additional mechanism to support "policy making...built on a fearless commitment to intellectual rigor, uncontaminated by commercial considerations, personal vested interests or peer group pressures."[6] L&I translates these mandatory HTA decisions into implementation policies operationalized in Washington's industrial insurance system.

As a second example, the Dr Robert Bree Collaborative of both public and private health care stakeholders has as its goals the identification and promotion of "strategies that improve patient health outcomes, health care service quality, and the affordability of health care."[16] The statutory mandate for the Bree Collaborative requires the analysis and identification of evidence-based best practices, which it translates into evidence-based practice recommendations.[17] These recommendations have recently resulted in efforts to improve the quality of low back pain care,[18] and in the development of a warranty bundle for lumbar fusion surgery.[19,20]

AGENCY REGULATORY AUTHORITY

Among L&I's core roles as an executive state agency is rule writing: the public and transparent process by which the legislative intent of statutes is translated into the clarifying details of the Washington Administrative Codes (WACs). These WACs define how those statutes will be implemented. The rules that result from this process have the force of law, and must comport with the underlying statutes. In this manner the same evidence-oriented mandate that exists in authorizing statutes also infuses many of the rules L&I develops. For example, WAC 296-20-02704 incorporates specific details about how scientific evidence is incorporated into agency medical coverage decisions.[21] Administrative code is also used to define how the department expects clinical evidence be used by providers to inform clinical decision making. One example, WAC 296-20-03070, proscribes the use of opioids in the absence of clinically meaningful improvement in function, which is a requirement for authorization of ongoing opioid prescriptions.[22,23]

THE JUDICIAL SYSTEM AND EVIDENCE-BASED POLICY

Precedential decisions from the judicial system may also directly influence L&I activity, touching at times on the evidence-based policies and decisions L&I produces. For example, interpretation and guidance articulated in Dennis v. Department of Labor and Industries (1987) continues to inform the day-to-day decisions L&I makes on the adjudication of occupational disease claims, and shapes agency policy on occupational diseases.[24]

AGENCY EXECUTIVE POLICY AUTHORITY

This combination of statute, administrative code, and judicial oversight establishes both the authority and boundaries of agency executive authority to implement industrial insurance policy. Consistent with the design of these democratic processes, L&I exercises its executive authority in a manner that respects the agency's role as a public health institution responsible to its principal public business and labor stake-holders, and honors its commitment to process transparency.

Simone Javaher's[25] discussion of treatment guideline development and evaluation speaks to both the transparency and manner in which evidence is incorporated into the work of Washington's Industrial Insurance Medical Advisory Committee (IIMAC). IIMAC is but 1 of several committees on which L&I relies to incorporate evidence from original research and public input to establish policy for the citizens of Washington. The Health Technology Clinical Committee and Bree Collaborative are other examples.

Evidence from original medical literature is similarly used by the Industrial Insurance Chiropractic Advisory Committee, which is charged with advising L&I "on matters related to the provision of safe, effective, and cost-effective chiropractic treatments for injured workers."[26,27]

Although the aims and membership of these groups differ according to the policy needs they support, these bodies share in common (1) transparent processes with meetings open to the public, (2) opportunities for public input, and (3) a statutory expectation to include scientific evidence into the work product.

Such public input, in conjunction with strong support and leadership from agency executives, is key to L&I's success at incorporating original research into the public policies the agency implements.

DEPARTMENT OF LABOR AND INDUSTRIES–FUNDED RESEARCH

The Washington laws governing industrial insurance also provide a statutory obligation that there "be constructed and maintained at the University of Washington an occupational and environmental research facility in the school of medicine having as its objects and purposes testing, research, training, teaching, consulting and service in the fields of industrial and occupational medicine and health, the prevention of industrial and occupational disease among workers, the promotion and protection of safer working environments and dissemination of the knowledge and information acquired from such objects and purposes."[28] This source of funding, supplemented by other grants, has also been the source of more than 20 years of outcomes research that has informed the agency's evidence-based policies.

To develop evidence-based policy L&I also relies in part on direct funding of research of import to the agency's mission. The Safety and Health Investment Projects Grant Program[29] is designed to reduce long-term disability and to support the development or implementation of ideas that promote return to work, or prevent fatalities, injuries, or illnesses at work. The products funded through this competitive grant mechanism are placed into the public domain and made available to the public, such as through posting to the L&I Web site.[30] Funds are paid for directly from the industrial insurance medical aid fund. Grants are reviewed in conjunction with a statutory advisory committee.[31]

Thus, both by statute and historical practice, L&I staff maintain close connections with the occupational health research community, in particular with the University of Washington. The L&I medical director maintains an appointment at the University of Washington, thereby not only sustaining the research relationships that promote academic inquiry directly responsive to Washington's occupational policy needs but also directly overseeing research projects relevant to agency policy activity. Responding to the epidemic of prescription opioid–related morbidity and mortality is a particularly salient example of the kind of research/policy integration that has resulted from such arrangements, and that permit L&I, along with the other Washington State agencies and medical directors, to implement the evidence-based policies needed to protect the public's health.[32]

Washington's Centers for Occupational Health and Education, described later, are another example of a strategically important population-level intervention born out of collaboration between L&I and occupational health researchers. The success of the initial pilot has justified expanding implementation to increase the number of workers who may access this intervention, aimed primarily at reducing long-term disability among injured workers.[33]

DEPARTMENT OF LABOR AND INDUSTRIES PILOT TESTING

L&I often uses the pilot project environment to help determine effectiveness of policy, to provide both financial and nonfinancial incentives for improving the industrial insurance system, and to make the changes necessary to piloted interventions to promote success before widespread implementation. Recent examples include determining that central administration of graded activity coaching (an intervention designed to promote recovery through activity) reached more workers than provider-based administration.[34] In addition, with L&I's current functional recovery pilot, the agency is determining how best to present providers with the information they require to address the needs of workers who are identified as being at high risk of developing long-term disability.[35]

Washington's Centers of Occupational Health and Education (COHE) also started as a pilot project to provide both financial and nonfinancial incentives to deliver occupational health best practices. After an analysis of the pilot project determined that COHEs were associated with reduced days of disability, and ultimately costs,[36] additional COHEs were established by the legislature.[37] There are now 6 COHEs in Washington, and expansion continues because of their strategic role in supporting disability prevention in Washington.[38]

REAL-TIME EVIDENCE ASSESSMENT

L&I's Ebola Virus Exposure and Disease Policy[39] for the state fund was developed internally under time-limited circumstances and without going through a statutory committee or complete systematic review. L&I's policy process nevertheless remained responsive to the needs of the public on this emerging issue and the agency ensured an institutional commitment to covered workers to restore income lost as a consequence of a work-related exposure to Ebola. By incorporating by reference the Centers for Disease Control and Prevention case definition of Ebola virus disease, and by relying on regularly updated state or federal criteria for establishing medical necessity for restrictions of movement, the policy remained true to known medical science concerning Ebola infection and transmission, while permitting the flexibility for criteria and definitions to evolve according to the need for health officials to protect the public, including Washington's workers. Policies such as this reflect how L&I "balance[s] gold standard systematic reviews with pragmatic, rapid reviews that gain in timeliness and accessibility what they lose in depth and detail."[4]

The complexity of certain policy questions do not require a full systematic review with a statutory committee, but the agency develops policies in such circumstances that still benefit from an internal culture that values the inclusion of original research as evidence where it exists, and has staff with the analytical skills needed to evaluate other, potentially unpublished, sources of information, such as agency administrative data.

SUMMARY

The experience at L&I of incorporating evidence into policies reflects many of the observations made in the literature that distinguishes the use of evidence for individual clinical encounters from the needs of a population for whom policies are established. Characteristics of L&I's policy process structure and evidence-based culture are also identified in original literature discussing the needs and barriers of incorporating evidence into public policy. L&I considers an agency culture that values original medical research and systematic review, dedication to transparent and accountable public processes, statutory expectation to incorporate evidence into policy, sustenance of relationships with the research community as well as research projects relevant to workers, and commitment to pilot testing and devotion of resources that translate innovative ideas into new public health interventions to all be essential to marshalling the public's resources and bringing to life a vision for Washington's industrial insurance system that is indelibly strengthened by the principles and research products of evidence-based medicine.

REFERENCES

1. Available at: http://apps.leg.wa.gov/RCW/default.aspx?cite=51.04.010. Accessed May 25, 2015.
2. Evidence-Based Medicine Working Group. Evidence-based medicine. A new approach to teaching the practice of medicine. JAMA 1992;268(17):2420.
3. Sackett DL, Rosenberg WM, Gray JA, et al. Evidence based medicine: What it is and what it isn't. BMJ 1996;312(7023):71–2.
4. Greenhalgh T, Howick J, Maskrey N, Evidence Based Medicine Renaissance Group. Evidence based medicine: a movement in crisis? BMJ 2014;348: g3725.
5. Rütten A. Evidence-based policy revisited: orientation towards the policy process and a public health policy science. Int J Public Health 2012;57(3):455–7.
6. Boaz A, Grayson L, Levitt R, et al. Does evidence-based policy work? Learning from the UK experience. Evidence & Policy 2008;4(2):233.
7. Bartlett W. Obstacles to evidence-based policy-making in the EU enlargement countries: the case of skills policies. Soc Policy Adm 2013;47(4):451.
8. Solesbury W. Evidence based policy: whence it came and where it's going. ESRC UK Centre for evidence based policy and practice. England: Queen Mary University of London; 2001.
9. Moseley C, Kleinert H, Sheppard-Jones K, et al. Using research evidence to inform public policy decisions. Intellect Dev Disabil 2013;51(5):412–22.
10. Hall AC, Butterworth J, Winsor J, et al. Pushing the employment agenda: case study research of high performing states in integrated employment. Intellect Dev Disabil 2007;45(3):182–98.
11. Oliver K, Lorenc T, Innvaer S. New directions in evidence-based policy research: a critical analysis of the literature. Health Res Policy Syst 2014;12:34.
12. Orton L, Lloyd-Williams F, Taylor-Robinson D, et al. The use of research evidence in public health decision making processes: systematic review. PLoS one 2011; 6(7):e21704.
13. Available at: http://apps.leg.wa.gov/RCW/default.aspx?cite=70.14.100. Accessed May 25, 2015.
14. Wang D, Liu TC. Prescription benchmarks for Washington. Cambridge (MA): Workers Compensation Research Institute; 2011.

15. Available at: http://www.hca.wa.gov/hta/Pages/about.aspx. Accessed May 25, 2015.

16. Available at: http://www.breecollaborative.org/about/. Accessed May 25, 2015.

17. Available at: http://apps.leg.wa.gov/RCW/default.aspx?cite=70.250.050. Accessed May 25, 2015.

18. Available at: http://www.breecollaborative.org/wp-content/uploads/spine_lbp.pdf. Accessed May 25, 2015.

19. Available at: http://www.breecollaborative.org/wp-content/uploads/Lumbar-Fusion-Warranty-Final-14-09.pdf. Accessed May 25, 2015.

20. Available at: http://www.breecollaborative.org/wp-content/uploads/Lumbar-Fusion-Bundle-Final-14-09.pdf. Accessed May 25, 2015.

21. Available at: http://apps.leg.wa.gov/WAC/default.aspx?cite=296-20-02704. Accessed May 25, 2015.

22. Available at: http://apps.leg.wa.gov/WAC/default.aspx?cite=296-20-03070. Accessed May 25, 2015.

23. Available at: http://apps.leg.wa.gov/WAC/default.aspx?cite=296-20-01002. Accessed May 25, 2015.

24. 109 Wn.2d 467, 745 P.2d 1295.

25. Javaher SP. Guideline development process in a public workers' compensation system. Phys Med Rehabil Clin N Am 2015;26(3):427–34.

26. Available at: http://www.lni.wa.gov/ClaimsIns/Providers/ProjResearchComm/IICAC/default.asp. Accessed May 25, 2015.

27. Available at: http://apps.leg.wa.gov/RCW/default.aspx?cite=51.36.150. Accessed May 25, 2015.

28. Available at: http://apps.leg.wa.gov/RCW/default.aspx?cite=28B.20.450. Accessed May 25, 2015.

29. Available at: http://lni.wa.gov/SAFETY/GRANTSPARTNERSHIPS/SHIP/DEFAULT.ASP. Accessed May 25, 2015.

30. Available at: http://lni.wa.gov/safety/GrantsPartnerships/SHIP/Grants.asp. Accessed May 25, 2015.

31. Available at: http://apps.leg.wa.gov/WAC/default.aspx?cite=296-900-17520. Accessed May 25, 2015.

32. Franklin GM, American Academy of Neurology. Opioids for chronic noncancer pain: A position paper of the American Academy of Neurology. Neurology 2014;83(14):1277–84.

33. Wickizer TM, Franklin G, Plaeger-Brockway R, et al. Improving the quality of workers' compensation health care delivery: The Washington State Occupational Health Services Project. Milbank Q 2001;79(1):5–33.

34. Available at: http://www.lni.wa.gov/ClaimsIns/Providers/Reforms/EmergingBP/Coaching.asp. Accessed May 25, 2015.

35. Available at: http://www.lni.wa.gov/ClaimsIns/Providers/Reforms/EmergingBP/FuncRecover.asp. Accessed May 25, 2015.

36. Wickizer T. Centers of occupational health and education: Final report on outcomes from the initial cohort of injured workers, 2003–2005. Seattle, Washington: University of Washington; 2007.

37. Substitute senate bill 5801, 2011-2012.

38. Available at: http://www.lni.wa.gov/ClaimsIns/Providers/ProjResearchComm/OHS/default.asp. Accessed May 25, 2015.

39. Available at: http://lni.wa.gov/ClaimsIns/Providers/TreatingPatients/ByCondition/Ebola.asp. Accessed May 25, 2015.

Application and Outcomes of Treatment Guidelines in a Utilization Review Program

Hal Stockbridge, MD, MPH[a,b,*], Nikki d'Urso, RN[a]

KEYWORDS

- Treatment guideline • Clinical practice guideline • Workers' compensation
- Utilization review • Utilization management • Cost containment • Quality of care
- Clinical outcomes

KEY POINTS

- The value and impact of treatment guidelines in improving outcomes for patients and controlling costs is significant.
- Incorporating evidence-based guidelines into a structured utilization review (UR) program is crucial for success.
- Most requests should be reviewed prospectively.
- Substantial return on investment can be achieved, particularly for procedures with high variation or questions of appropriateness.

INTRODUCTION

The value and impact of treatment guidelines in improving outcomes for patients and controlling costs is significantly enhanced in Washington state workers' compensation by incorporating the guidelines into a structured UR program.

This article briefly describes (1) how the Washington State Department of Labor and Industries (L&I) UR program uses treatment guidelines and (2) the impact of the UR program on costs and outcomes.

THE WASHINGTON UTILIZATION REVIEW PROCESS

Since the 1980s, the Washington workers' compensation UR process has supported the purchase of proper and necessary care for injured workers. UR is required for all inpatient services, all spinal injections, advanced imaging (MRI studies of the spine,

Conflicts of Interest: None.
[a] Washington State Department of Labor and Industries, PO Box 44321, Olympia, WA 98504-4321, USA; [b] University of Washington, Seattle, WA, USA
* Corresponding author.
E-mail address: Stoh235@Lni.wa.gov

Phys Med Rehabil Clin N Am 26 (2015) 445–452
http://dx.doi.org/10.1016/j.pmr.2015.04.011
1047-9651/15/$ – see front matter Published by Elsevier Inc.

pmr.theclinics.com

upper and lower extremities, and brain MRI and computed tomography [CT] studies for headaches), physical and occupational therapy after the 24th visit, and selected outpatient intervention services. The UR process compares requests for medical services with medical treatment guidelines that are deemed appropriate for such services and includes the preparation of a recommendation based on that comparison. The UR program applies only to claims that are adjudicated by the State Fund (not self-insured employers). The program applies to both physicians and facilities. L&I contracts with Qualis Health for UR. Qualis Health is a health care consulting organization, with headquarters in Seattle, Washington, and regional offices located in Alabama, Alaska, California, Idaho, and the District of Columbia.

Providers requesting authorization are asked to refer to L&I's Medical Treatment Guidelines for information on what specific clinical information is required for selected procedures. (For details on L&I's Medical Treatment Guidelines see links below.) Qualis Health uses the Department's Medical Treatment Guidelines as the basis for their recommendations. When there are no Department Medical Treatment Guidelines available, Qualis Health uses InterQual proprietary criteria. An initial clinical review is conducted by a registered nurse or physical therapist. If it does not meet guidelines or criteria, it is referred for physician review. If the physician reviewer is unable to recommend approval, the requesting physician has the opportunity to discuss the case with a Qualis physician. A re-review option is available with a practicing matched specialty provider. Qualis Health recommendations are then sent to the L&I claim manager. The claim manager reviews the information and recommendation made by Qualis Health and then decides whether to authorize or deny the request.

A streamlined authorization process was created for what are called Group A providers. Providers may be eligible to become Group A providers if they have 100% UR approval recommendations when they performed 10 or more reviews during a 1-year review period. Group A providers are not required to submit clinical information, chart notes, or diagnostic reports to Qualis Health for most outpatient surgeries. They are required to submit a form with the planned procedure, description and current procedural terminology (CPT) codes, place of service, date or anticipated date of service, and office contact name and phone number. However, even Group A providers must follow the full clinic review process for all spine procedures and other complex surgeries. Retrospective audit of 20% of cases is completed on all Group A providers to ensure continued compliance with the guidelines. All providers are reviewed annually to determine Group A eligibility.

For some reviews, Qualis Health provides Web-based UR, which allows providers to submit and review request status online and to complete questionnaires online that can affect the request status. By using a combination of questionnaires and checklists along with Web-based submission, the cost of UR can be reduced and the turnaround time for authorizations can be substantially reduced.

For advanced imaging authorization, the department requires requesting providers to use a Web-based system; this applies to MRI of the spine, upper extremity, and lower extremity and brain MRI or CT of the head due to headache. This requirement was put in place because the Washington Legislature passed a law in 2009 (engrossed substitute house bill [ESHB] 2105, Chapter 258) that directed the State to convene an Advanced Imaging Management Work Group. State agencies were directed to implement the Work Group recommendations.

More detail about the Washington UR program can be found at: http://lni.wa.gov/ClaimsIns/Providers/AuthRef/UtilReview.

More detail about L&I's Medical Treatment Guidelines can be found at: http://lni.wa.gov/ClaimsIns/Providers/TreatingPatients/TreatGuide.

IMPACT OF GUIDELINES AND UTILIZATION REVIEW

The financial impact of the implementation of guidelines in the Washington UR program is considerable. Based on quarterly data from 2014, the L&I UR program produced annual gross savings of an estimated $14,925,386; costs of the UR program were $7,405,563; net savings were $7,519,824; and the return on investment was approximately $2.00. Here is a breakdown of the numbers:

- Inpatient cases: Estimated annual savings $3,920,000; cost of review $1,113,840; net savings $2,806,160; return on investment $3.52
- Outpatient cases: Estimated annual savings $1,882,492; cost of review $1,026,000; net savings $856,492; return on investment $1.83
- Outpatient discography cases: Estimated annual savings $18,400; cost of review $2880; net savings $15,520; return on investment $6.39
- Outpatient physical medicine cases: Estimated annual savings $4,411,095; cost of review $2,334,548; net savings $2,076,547; return on investment $1.89
- Imaging cases: Estimated annual savings $2,831,159; cost of review $1,233,720; net savings $1,597,439; return on investment $2.29
- Spinal injection cases: Estimated annual savings $1,862,240; cost of review $1,233,720; net savings $628,520; return on investment $1.51

The aforementioned numbers likely underestimate the cost savings. These savings reports reflect denials of requested services that were found not to meet guidelines. But when other measures are considered, a bigger impact is observed. Data suggest that there would have been many requests for authorization that were not submitted because the provider was aware of the guidelines and understood that a request would not meet guidelines. For example, when a new guideline is created or a guideline is revised, efforts are made to assess the impact of the changes on patient outcomes and costs. Spinal injections performed on an outpatient basis were affected by a guideline issued in 2012. L&I studied a baseline number of spinal injections before implementing UR and compared it with the current numbers. Data from September 2012 through September 2014 suggest that the number of spinal injections has decreased by 40%. Similarly, after UR for advanced imaging was implemented in 2010, costs dropped dramatically. Between 2009 and 2013, total costs for advanced imaging dropped from $30 million to $14 million. The annual UR cost is roughly $1 million. Clearly, the return on investment has been significant. Thus, the impact of evidence-based UR is both direct, specific to denial rates of known requests, and indirect, related to an important sentinel effect of implementation.

The impact on quality of care and clinical outcomes from the UR program includes an overarching effect from using evidence-based standards of care to encourage providers to use best practices and to perform procedures when appropriate for given clinical circumstances. As described elsewhere in this issue, L&I's treatment guidelines represent a thorough review of the scientific medical literature by recognized clinical experts from the University of Washington and other medical institutions and by internal epidemiology staff. They are evidence based, along with a process based on consensus among the clinical experts participating in a statutorily established medical advisory committee. The process is transparent and includes public input. The guidelines are widely disseminated and are available through the National Guideline Clearinghouse (see www.guideline.gov). With this background, it is likely that clinical outcomes are improved when the UR process results in avoiding unnecessary procedures and authorizing procedures when they are likely to be of benefit to the injured worker.

It can be difficult to quantify effects on quality of care. One potential proxy measure of the value of the UR program in Washington workers' compensation in achieving high-quality care is the low number of denials overturned on appeal. A small number of denied authorizations are appealed. Quarterly average re-reviews are 55. The re-review process includes a second review by a matched specialty provider. L&I's current re-review rate is 2.2%, and 83% of those reviews have determination to uphold the original recommendation.

Little research has been done on the impact of UR on cost or quality of care. Although the focus of this article is on the Washington UR program, studies in Washington and other states have provided some limited data on the impact of UR, with varying results. Here is a sample of the published literature relating to UR:

- A study in the late 1980s analyzed Aetna's UR customers compared with a representative sample of its customers who had no UR. Statistical adjustments were made for the utilization management status, employee demographics, plan benefits, group size, year effects, and seasonality. The data suggested that UR reduced overall medical expenses by 4.4% and inpatient expenses by 8.1%, largely by reducing length of stay.[1]
- A study was conducted by the Columbia University in 1989. New York City and its unions temporarily replaced actual UR with sham review for half the participants in the city's fee-for-service health insurance plan. The results were mixed, with a conclusion that the UR program probably had little effect.[2]
- A study published in 1997 analyzed the effects of guidelines for elective lumbar fusion as part of its inpatient UR program. Discharge data from the Comprehensive Hospital Abstract Reporting System were used to identify lumbar surgical cases. After November 1988, when the guidelines went into effect, the state rates for fusion operations declined 33%, whereas rates for nonfusion operations essentially were unchanged. The sharpest decline corresponded in time to implementation of the guidelines. Before the initiation of L&I guidelines, the proportion of fusions among L&I patients was higher than among non-L&I patients. The opposite was true by the end of 1992, and the L&I proportion decreased more rapidly than the non-L&I proportion. The researchers concluded that the data suggest that the L&I lumbar fusion surgery criteria and reimbursement standards implemented in 1988 contributed to a decline in rates of performing that procedure, with a sentinel effect on statewide fusion operation rates, not just in workers' compensation. The UR aspect of the guidelines as well as the process of involving surgeons in the preparation and dissemination of guidelines also may have been contributory.[3]
- A 1999 study analyzed a study population residing primarily in the South and Midwest. It analyzed 11,785 UR reviews performed on workers' compensation patients from 1991 through 1993. The investigators concluded: "The long-run value of utilization management (UM) as an approach to containing costs and improving quality within the workers' compensation system remains an unanswered question. The general perception among medical professionals and administrators is that UM, as practiced, is burdensome, inefficient, and clinically unscientific. We believe that these weaknesses can, and should, be addressed. As more and better treatment outcome information becomes available, it will be possible to improve UM review protocols by linking the review criteria more closely to current knowledge of medical outcomes and clinical epidemiology. UM is burdensome and inefficient because it relies on a global 'one size fits all' approach to the performance of review screening. It is time that more clinically

sophisticated, targeted approaches be developed that could better accomplish the objectives of cost containment and quality improvement, at lower expense."[4]

- A study analyzed an orthopedic UR program in Washington workers' compensation in the early 1990s. The outcomes of back and neck injury claims (primarily sprains and strains) filed in the 2 months after the program was fully operational were compared with 2 comparable groups of claims from the same base population filed before the program's availability. The study found no difference between subjects and controls with respect to work-loss days, rate of claim closure, or permanent impairment. This quality-based program, used as an adjunct to claims management, failed to improve outcomes. However, this program was based on use of an analytics program to send data on potential red flags to claims staff, with the outcomes reliant on claims adjudicators' action. This program did not depend on review and denial/acceptance of specific procedures.[5]

- Another study analyzed a UR program in Washington workers' compensation, which used guidelines developed collaboratively with the state medical association. These guidelines dealt with 10 areas: medical back hospital admissions, lumbar arthrodesis, lumbar laminectomy, thoracic outlet syndrome surgery, cervical laminectomy, knee surgery, shoulder surgery, ankle/foot surgery, lumbar MRI, and carpal tunnel surgery. From 1993 through 1998, a total of 100,005 UR reviews were conducted, half of which used the guideline-based review criteria. The overall denial rate for the guideline-based reviews was 7.3%. The highest denial rates were for thoracic outlet syndrome surgery (19.1%) and lumbar fusion (17.7%). The investigators concluded that the use of guideline-based UR protocols may improve the effectiveness of UR as a tool to identify potentially inappropriate care.[6]

- There are a variety of treatment guidelines used by UR programs across the United States. A report on the process of selecting workers' compensation treatment guidelines in California described screening criteria using an internationally accepted tool (the Appraisal of Guidelines Research and Evaluation Instrument) to evaluate the technical quality of these guideline sets. The 5 guideline sets meeting the criteria were Clinical Guidelines by the American Academy of Orthopedic Surgeons, American College of Occupational and Environmental Medicine Occupational Medicine Practice Guidelines, Optimal Treatment Guidelines (Intra-Corp), McKesson/InterQual Care Management Criteria and Clinical Evidence Summary (McKesson), and Official Disability Guidelines. The researchers conclude that selecting mandatory workers' compensation guidelines should involve careful planning and a transparent, well-defined process.[7]

- A study of the Wisconsin workers' compensation system analyzed health outcomes and compared Wisconsin with 10 other states (California, Tennessee, Florida, North Carolina, Maryland, Texas, Connecticut, Michigan, Pennsylvania, and Massachusetts). In Wisconsin, UR is not required and there are no UR regulations. Among the 10 comparison states studied, UR is not required in Connecticut, Maryland, or Pennsylvania. The other 7 states (California, Florida, Massachusetts, Michigan, North Carolina, Tennessee, and Texas) all require UR. In 2009, researchers conducted interviews with workers injured in 2006. The interviews assessed improvement in health status from injury to interview, using the Short Form Health Survey (SF-12), which was developed for the Medical Outcomes Study, a multiyear study of patients with chronic conditions. The study found the following:
  ○ The median time from injury to first substantial return to work (as of 2.5 years postinjury) was lowest for Wisconsin (6 weeks) and highest for California (12 weeks).

○ The increase in the SF-12 score from the week after injury to the time of the interview was third best in Wisconsin (Pennsylvania and Massachusetts were better). The worst was California.

○ The percentage who were "somewhat" or "very" satisfied with overall health care was highest for Wisconsin at 89%. (California was lowest at 70%.)

This study seems to suggest that a system such as Wisconsin's can achieve good outcomes without a UR program.[8]

• The Workers Compensation Research Institute, based in Cambridge, Massachusetts, compiled a national inventory of cost containment programs in workers' compensation in 2013. It found that many states have no requirement for UR (such as Arizona, Colorado, Connecticut, Idaho, Maryland, New York, Ohio, Oregon, and Pennsylvania). In some states, only certified review organizations are authorized to perform UR functions (such as Arkansas, Illinois, Maine, Massachusetts, Mississippi, Texas, and Washington). In some states, the claims that are subject to UR include all inpatient hospitalizations and planned invasive surgery (such as Alabama, Kentucky, North Dakota, and Washington). In some states, use of treatment guidelines is mandatory. Examples of states where it is mandatory include California, Colorado, Florida, Massachusetts, Minnesota, New York, Ohio, Texas, and Washington. Examples of states where it is not mandatory include Connecticut, Illinois, Michigan, Oregon, and Pennsylvania.[9]

• A study published in 2014 compared California and Washington State with respect to population-level effects of lumbar fusion policy differences on utilization, costs, and safety. Washington State's workers' compensation program requires imaging confirmation of instability and limits initial fusions to a single level. In contrast, California requires coverage if a second opinion supports surgery, allows initial multilevel fusion, and provides additional reimbursement for surgical implants. The study identified workers' compensation patients (n = 4628) in California and Washington using the Agency for Healthcare Research and Quality's State Inpatient Databases, 2008–2009. Outcome measures included repeat lumbar spine surgery, all-cause readmission, life-threatening complications, wound problems, device complications, and costs. Analysis showed that California patients were more likely than those in Washington to undergo fusion for controversial indications, such as nonspecific back pain (28% vs 21%) and disc herniation (37% vs 21%), as opposed to spinal stenosis (6% vs 15%) and spondylolisthesis (25% vs 41%). California had higher adjusted risk for reoperation (relative risk [RR] 2.28; 95% confidence interval [CI], 2.27–2.29), wound problems (RR, 2.64; 95% CI, 2.62–2.65), device complications (RR, 2.49; 95% CI, 2.38–2.61), and life-threatening complications (RR, 1.31; 95% CI, 1.31–1.31). Hospital costs for the index procedure were greater in California ($49,430) than in Washington ($40,114).[10]

SUMMARY

In summary, before the UR program was in place in Washington's workers' compensation system, numerous diagnostic and therapeutic procedures were performed unnecessarily, with both potential and real detrimental effects on patients. As described in other articles in this issue, procedures such as cervical fusion and surgery for thoracic outlet syndrome often have very poor outcomes, especially in workers' compensation populations. To the extent that a UR program can help assure that such procedures are only performed when the patient is likely to benefit, UR programs may contribute in a major way to improved quality of care. The authors believe that the methods used at the Washington State Department of L&I reflect the best practices in UR. The vendor, Qualis Health, relies on criteria established by national UR standards groups, such as URAC (https://www.urac.org/).

REFERENCES

1. Khandker RK, Manning WG. The impact of utilization review on costs and utilization. Dev Health Econ Public Policy 1992;1:47–62.
2. Rosenberg SN, Allen DR, Handte JS, et al. Effect of utilization review in a fee-for-service health insurance plan. N Engl J Med 1995;333(20):1326–30.
3. Elam K, Taylor V, Ciol MA, et al. Impact of a worker's compensation practice guideline on lumbar spine fusion in Washington State. Med Care 1997;35(5):417–24.
4. Wickizer TM, Lessler D, Franklin G. Controlling workers' compensation medical care use and costs through utilization management. J Occup Environ Med 1999;41:625–31.
5. Battié MC, Fulton-Kehoe D, Franklin G. The effects of a medical care utilization review program on back and neck injury claims. J Occup Environ Med 2002; 44(4):365–71.
6. Wickizer TM, Franklin G, Gluck JV, et al. Improving quality through identifying inappropriate care: the use of guideline-based utilization review protocols in the Washington state workers' compensation system. J Occup Environ Med 2004;46(3):198–204.
7. Harber P, Wynn BO, Lim YW, et al. Selection of workers' compensation treatment guidelines: California experience. J Occup Environ Med 2008;50(11):1282–92.
8. Belton SE. How have worker outcomes and medical costs changed in Wisconsin? Cambridge (UK): Massachusetts: Workers Compensation Research Institute; 2010.
9. Ramona PT. Workers' compensation medical cost containment: a national inventory, 2013. The Workers Compensation Research Institute, Cambridge (UK): Massachusetts: Workers Compensation Research Institute; 2013. p. WC-13-02.
10. Martin BI, Franklin GM, Deyo RA, et al. How do coverage policies influence practice patterns, safety, and cost of initial lumbar fusion surgery? A population-based comparison of workers' compensation systems. Spine J 2014;14(7): 1237–46.

FURTHER READINGS

Bernacki EJ, Tsai SP. Ten years' experience using an integrated workers' compensation management system to control workers' compensation costs. J Occup Environ Med 2003;45:508–16.
Feldstein PJ, Wickizer TM, Wheeler JR. Private cost containment: the effects of utilization review programs on health care use and expenditures. N Engl J Med 1988; 318(20):1310–4.
Nuckolls TK, Wynn BO, Lim Y, et al. Evaluating medical treatment guideline sets for injured workers in California. Santa Monica, CA: RAND Corporation; 2005. Available at: http://www.rand.org/pubs/monographs/MG400.
Wickizer TM, Wheeler JR, Feldstein PJ. Does utilization review reduce unnecessary hospital care and contain costs? Med Care 1989;27(6):632–47.
Wickizer TM, Feldstein PJ, Wheeler JR, et al. Reducing hospital use and expenditures through utilization review. Findings from an outcome evaluation. Qual Assur Util Rev 1990;5(3):80–5.

Wickizer TM. Effect of hospital utilization review on medical expenditures in selected diagnostic areas: an exploratory study. Am J Public Health 1991;81(4):482–4.

Wickizer TM, Wheeler JR, Feldstein PJ. Have hospital inpatient cost containment programs contributed to the growth in outpatient expenditures? Analysis of the substitution effect associated with hospital utilization review. Med Care 1991; 29(5):442–51.

Wickizer TM. The effects of utilization review on hospital use and expenditures: a covariance analysis. Health Serv Res 1992;27(1):103–21.

Wickizer TM. Controlling outpatient medical equipment costs through utilization management. Med Care 1995;33(4):383–91.

Guideline for Prescribing Opioids to Treat Pain in Injured Workers

Jaymie Mai, PharmD[a], Gary Franklin, MD, MPH[a,b,*], David Tauben, MD[c]

KEYWORDS

- Opioids • Workers' compensation • Injured workers • Chronic pain • Acute pain
- Surgical pain • Addiction

KEY POINTS

- Effective use of opioids must result in clinically meaningful improvement in function (CMIF). Continuing to prescribe opioids in the absence of CMIF or after the development of a severe adverse outcome is not medically necessary care in workers' compensation.
- Chronic opioid therapy should not be prescribed in the presence of current substance use disorder (excluding nicotine) or a history of opioid use disorder, and the prescriber should use caution if there is a history of other substance use disorders.
- Use of chronic opioid therapy requires regular monitoring and documentation, such as screening for risk of comorbid conditions with validated tools, checking the Prescription Monitoring Program database, assessing function, and administering random urine drug tests.
- Patients on chronic opioid therapy who are undergoing elective surgery are more likely to encounter difficulty with postoperative pain control.
- Opioids should be discontinued if treatment has not resulted in CMIF, or the worker has experienced a severe adverse outcome or overdose event.

INTRODUCTION

The Washington State Agency Medical Director's Group (AMDG) originally published a guideline for safely prescribing chronic opioid therapy (COT) in 2007 with an update in 2010 (http://www.agencymeddirectors.wa.gov/opioiddosing.asp). Between 2011 and 2012, the Industrial Insurance Medical Advisory Committee and its subcommittee on

[a] Washington State Department of Labor and Industries, Olympia, WA, USA; [b] Department of Environmental Health, Neurology and Health Services, University of Washington, Seattle, WA, USA; [c] Division of Pain Medicine, Anesthesia and Pain Medicine, University of Washington Medical Center, University of Washington, Seattle, WA, USA
* Corresponding author. Occupational Epidemiology and Health Outcomes Program, 130 Nickerson, Suite 212, Seattle, WA 98109, USA.
E-mail address: fral235@lni.wa.gov

Phys Med Rehabil Clin N Am 26 (2015) 453–465
http://dx.doi.org/10.1016/j.pmr.2015.04.005
1047-9651/15/$ – see front matter © 2015 Elsevier Inc. All rights reserved.

pmr.theclinics.com

chronic noncancer pain developed this guideline as a supplement to provide information specific to treating injured workers. It is based on the best available clinical and scientific evidence from a systematic review of the literature and a consensus of expert opinion.

Opioids are commonly prescribed for routine musculoskeletal injuries such as sprains and strains, despite a lack of evidence to support this practice. Studies have shown that opioids are being prescribed at higher doses, corresponding to a dramatic increase in accidental deaths.[1–3] In addition, chronic opioid use is associated with increased risk for other nonfatal adverse outcomes such as nonfatal overdose, dependence, addiction, and endocrine dysfunction. In some cases, the use of opioids for work-related injuries may actually increase the likelihood of disability. Because of the uncertainty of long-term efficacy with opioids, but clear evidence of harms, preventing the next group of workers from developing chronic disability and other opioid-related harms is a key objective of this guideline. The AMDG Guideline and this guideline represent the best practices and universal precautions necessary to safely and effectively prescribe opioids to treat injured workers with chronic noncancer pain.[4] These guidelines are intended for use by health care providers when prescribing opioids and as coverage policy for the department and insurers.

OPIOID USE IN WORKERS' COMPENSATION
Prevalence

Over the past decade, there has been a dramatic increase in the use of opioids to treat chronic noncancer pain. Among the workers' compensation population nationally, the prevalence of opioid use is approximately 32%.[5] In Washington, 42% of workers with compensable back injuries received an opioid prescription in the first year after injury, most often at the first medical visit for the injury. Sixteen percent of those workers were still receiving opioids 1 year after injury.[6]

Opioids are also being prescribed in stronger potencies and larger doses for musculoskeletal injuries.[2,5,7] The most potent class of opioids, schedule II, accounted for 43% of all opioid prescriptions in Washington workers' compensation in 2008, compared with 19% in 1996.[8] During this same timeframe, the average morphine equivalent dose (MED) of schedule II long-acting opioids increased from 88 mg/d to 132 mg/d.[2,8] The average dose remained relatively steady through 2008 and then declined, likely related to the publication of the AMDG Guideline.[9]

Impact on Recovery

In some cases, the use of opioids for work-related injuries may actually increase the likelihood of disability. Receiving more than a 1-week supply of opioids or 2 or more opioid prescriptions soon after an injury doubles a worker's risk of disability at 1 year after injury, compared with workers who do not receive opioids.[10] Other states have seen similar outcomes, including correlation between large-dose escalations and increasing duration of time loss.[2,11,12] Evidence-based guidelines on the management of acute low back pain recommend conservative initial therapies (eg, acetaminophen or nonsteroidal anti-inflammatory drugs [NSAIDs]) rather than opioids in almost all cases.[13,14]

Opioid-related Adverse Outcomes

Recent epidemiologic studies have shown that COT patients receiving greater than 100 mg/d MED have up to 9 times the risk of overdosing compared with those on 20 mg/d, and for every 7 overdoses, one was fatal.[15–17] These studies further showed that even at doses of 50 to 100 mg/d MED, risk was 2.2 to 4.6 times higher compared with doses less than 20 mg/d MED. In addition, COT is associated with significant risk of nonfatal adverse outcomes and the development of tolerance to its analgesic effects. The traditional prescribing practice was to use escalating doses to overcome this effect. However, evidence is accumulating that chronic, high-dose opioid use may lead to the development of abnormal pain sensitivity (opioid-induced hyperalgesia).[18] Dose escalation that does not improve pain and function can lead to increased risk for severe adverse outcomes. These adverse outcomes include inhibition of endogenous sex hormone production, neonatal abstinence syndrome, central sleep apnea, opioid use disorder (as defined in the Diagnostic and Statistical Manual of Mental Disorders 5 or DSM-5 at www.dsm5.org/Pages/Default.aspx), overdose, and death.

Measuring the Impact of Opioid Use

Beyond the acute phase, effective use of opioids should result in clinically meaningful improvement in function (CMIF). Providers should track function and pain on a regular basis, using the same validated instruments at each visit, to consistently determine the effect of opioid therapy. The department endorses the Two-Item Graded Chronic Pain Scale[19] as a quick, 2-question tool to track both function and pain when opioids are prescribed (see AMDG Guideline, Appendix C, at www.agencymeddirectors.wa. gov/Files/OpioidGdline.pdf).

CMIF is defined as an improvement in function of at least 30% as compared with the start of treatment or in response to a dose change.[20,21] A decrease in pain intensity in the absence of improved function is not considered CMIF.

Other validated instruments may also be used to measure functional improvement (see AMDG Guideline, Tools for Assessing Function and Pain at www. agencymeddirectors.wa.gov/Files/OpioidGdline.pdf). The American Chronic Pain Association has created a 10-item Quality-of-Life Scale for people with pain, which helps correlate the Graded Chronic Pain Scale with actual daily activities.[22] Use of the PROMIS Web-based tool (www.nihpromis.org/) may also be helpful in determining the effectiveness of COT. Ultimately, effective COT should result in improved work capacity or the ability to progress in vocational retraining.

Evaluation of clinically meaningful improvement should occur at the 3 following critical decision-making phases:

1. At the end of the acute phase (about 6 weeks following injury or surgery), to determine whether continued opioid therapy is warranted in the subacute phase.
2. At the end of the subacute phase (3 months following injury), to determine whether to prescribe COT.
3. Periodically during COT, to assess impact on function and risk of therapy.

Continuing to prescribe opioids in the absence of CMIF or after the development of a severe adverse outcome is not considered proper and necessary care in the workers' compensation system. In addition, the use of escalating doses to the point of developing opioid use disorder is not proper and necessary care.

OPIOID PRESCRIBING PRECAUTIONS
Opioid Use with Comorbid Substance Use or Mental Health Disorders

Managing pain in workers with complex medical conditions such as substance use disorder or a mental health condition can be a challenge. Research has shown that patients with substance use or psychiatric disorders, or both, are actually more likely than patients without these disorders to receive COT.[23] They are also more likely to have complications such as misuse, abuse, or overdose.[24,25] Adults with a history of depression, alcohol or other nonopioid drug abuse, or dependence are 3 to 5 times more likely to receive COT.[26] In addition, nicotine dependence is associated with a greater likelihood of using opioids and at higher doses.[27]

Among adults with chronic pain, COT use is increasing more rapidly in those with mental health and substance use disorders than in those without these diagnoses. These patients are also more likely to receive schedule II opioids, to receive opioids at higher dosage levels, and to be prescribed sedative-hypnotic medications on a chronic basis, than those without mental health or substance use disorders.[28]

High-risk COT prescribing practices (high opioid dose, extended COT duration, concurrent use of sedatives/hypnotics) are associated with increased risks of opioid overdose and serious fractures.[15,29] Unfortunately, patients who receive high-risk COT are also more likely to have high-risk characteristics, including younger age, history of substance abuse and mental disorder, and presence of opioid misuse.[30]

Because of the increased risk for adverse outcomes from the use of COT in patients with mental health disorders, such as borderline personality disorder, mood disorders (eg, depression, bipolar disorder, anxiety, posttraumatic stress disorder or PTSD), or psychotic disorders, providers should be cautious when prescribing COT for workers with these comorbid conditions. Furthermore, workers with current substance use disorders as defined by DSM (excluding nicotine) should not receive COT. Workers with a history of opioid use disorder should only receive COT under exceptional circumstances.

Drugs and Drug Combinations to Avoid

Do not use:
- Parenteral opioids in an outpatient setting
- Meperidine for chronic pain
- Methadone for acute or breakthrough pain
- Long-acting or extended-release opioids (eg, Oxycontin) for acute pain or postoperative pain in an opioid-naive worker

Use is not recommended:
- Carisoprodol (Soma)
- Any combination of opioids with benzodiazepines, sedative-hypnotics, or barbiturates. There may be specific indications for such combinations, such as the coexistence of spasticity. In such cases, a pain specialist consultation is strongly recommended. Consider alternatives such as tricyclic antidepressants or antihistamines to manage insomnia.

Use with caution:
- Over-the-counter acetaminophen with acetaminophen combination opioids (eg, Vicodin, Norco, Percocet, Endocet, Ultracet)
- Tramadol or meperidine in patients at risk for seizures or who are taking drugs that can cause seizures (eg, bupropion, serotonin reuptake inhibitors, tricyclic antidepressants)
- Methadone for pain (**Box 1**). Because of methadone's nonlinear pharmacokinetics, unpredictable clearance, and multiple drug-drug interactions, providers should use extreme caution when prescribing this drug for pain. Additional information is available at www.agencymeddirectors.wa.gov/opioiddosing.asp.

> **Box 1**
> **Prescribing methadone is complex. To prevent serious complications from methadone, prescribers should read and carefully follow the methadone (Dolophine) prescribing information at www.accessdata.fda.gov/scripts/cder/drugsatfda/index.cfm**
>
> Deaths, cardiac and respiratory, have been reported during initiation and conversion of pain patients to methadone treatment from treatment with other opioid agonists. It is critical to understand the pharmacokinetics of methadone when converting patients from other opioids.
>
> Respiratory depression is the chief hazard associated with methadone administration. Methadone's peak respiratory depressant effects typically occur later and persist longer than its peak analgesic effects, particularly in the early dosing period. These characteristics can contribute to cases of iatrogenic overdose, particularly during treatment initiation and dose titration.
>
> In addition, cases of QT interval prolongation and serious arrhythmia (torsades de pointes) have been observed during treatment with methadone. Most cases involve patients being treated for pain with large, multiple daily doses of methadone, although cases have been reported in patients receiving doses commonly used for maintenance treatment of opioid addiction.
>
> Methadone treatment for analgesic therapy in patients with acute or chronic pain should only be initiated if the potential analgesic or palliative care benefit of treatment with methadone is considered and outweighs the risks.

PRESCRIBING OPIOIDS FOR A WORK-RELATED INJURY OR OCCUPATIONAL DISEASE
Opioids in the Acute Phase (0–6 Weeks After Injury or Surgery)

In general, opioid use for acute pain should be reserved for after surgery, for the most severe pain (eg, pain scores ≥7), or when alternative treatments such as NSAIDs and nonpharmacologic therapies are ineffective. Evidence does not support the use of opioids as initial treatment of back sprain or other strains, but if they are prescribed, use should be limited to short term (eg, ≤ 14 days).

Pain intensity and pain interference should decrease during the acute phase as part of the natural course of recovery following surgery or most injuries. Resumption of pre-injury activities, such as return to work, should be expected during this period. If use in the acute phase (0–6 weeks) does not lead to improvements in pain and function of at least 30%, or to pain interference levels of 4 or less, continued opioid use is not warranted.

Preliminary data from the Washington state Prescription Monitoring Program (PMP) have suggested that substantial numbers of newly injured workers received opioids or other controlled substances in the 60 days before injury. For this reason, providers should check the PMP before prescribing opioids for new injuries or occupational diseases.

Providers should:
- Check the state's PMP (http://pdmpassist.org/content/state-pdmp-websites) with any initial opioid prescription for a new episode of pain.
- Obtain baseline measures of pain and pain interference (function) within 2 weeks of filing a claim.
- Help the worker set reasonable expectations about their recovery and return to work.
- Talk to the worker about safe storage and disposal of opioids and other controlled substances.

- Prescribe opioids in multiples of 7-day supply to reduce the incidence of supply ending on a weekend.
- Document CMIF and pain with treatment.
- Explore nonopioid strategies to treat pain, including early activation.
- Use urine drug tests (UDTs), the state's PMP, and other screening tools in the AMDG Guideline (www.agencymeddirectors.wa.gov/opioiddosing.asp) to ensure controlled substances history is consistent with prescribing record and worker's report.
- Determine preinjury use of controlled substances and help the worker understand that the insurer is not responsible for non-work-related treatment and conditions.
- Discontinue opioids after the acute pain episode if clinically meaningful improvements in function and pain have not been achieved.

Opioids in the Subacute Phase (Between 6 and 12 Weeks)

With some exceptions, resumption of preinjury activities such as return to work should be expected during this period. Use of activity diaries (http://www.agencymeddirectors.wa.gov/Files/ActivityDiary.pdf) is encouraged as a means of improving patient participation and investment in recovery. Nonpharmacologic treatments, such as cognitive-behavioral therapy, activity coaching, and graded exercise, are also encouraged.[13,31] If the injury is a sprain or strain, opioid use beyond the acute phase is rarely indicated.

If opioids are to be prescribed for longer than 6 weeks and with the exception of catastrophic injuries, the provider should perform the following best practices:

- Access the state's PMP to ensure that the controlled substance history is consistent with the prescribing record and worker's report.
- Document CMIF and pain with acute use.
- Screen worker for depression (eg, patient health questionnaire 9 (PHQ-9) or other validated tools) to identify potential comorbid conditions, which may impact response to opioid treatment. If the worker's history suggests PTSD, administer the 4-item PC-PTSD screen (www.integration.samhsa.gov/clinical-practice/PC-PTSD.pdf).
- Screen for opioid risk (eg, Opioid Risk Tool, screener and opioid assessment for patients with pain (SOAPP-R), diagnosis, intractability, risk, efficacy (DIRE), or CAGE-AID). If the worker has current substance use disorder (excluding nicotine) or a history of opioid use disorder, opioid use beyond the acute phase is rarely indicated.
- Administer a baseline UDT. If results reveal "red flags" such as the confirmed presence of cocaine, amphetamines, or alcohol, opioid use beyond the acute phase is not indicated (see AMDG Guideline, Appendix D at www.agencymeddirectors.wa.gov/Files/OpioidGdline.pdf). Unless cannabis use disorder is diagnosed, the presence of cannabis on a UDT does not preclude the use of opioids.
- Re-examine and consider discontinuation or taper of concurrent sedative-hypnotics or benzodiazepines.

During the subacute phase, providers should review the effects of opioid therapy on pain and function to determine whether opioid therapy should continue. Opioids should be discontinued during this phase if:

- There is no CMIF when compared with function measured during the acute phase.
- The treatment resulted in a severe adverse outcome.

- The worker has a current substance use disorder (excluding nicotine).
- The worker has a history of opioid use disorder (with rare exceptions).

Opioids in the Chronic Phase

If opioids are to be prescribed beyond 12 weeks after injury or after surgery, and with the exception of catastrophic injuries, the provider should document the following:

- CMIF (≥30%) has been established with opioid use in the acute or subacute phase.
- Failure of trials of reasonable alternatives to opioids.
- Signed treatment agreement (pain contract).
- A time-limited treatment plan, addressing whether COT is likely to improve the worker's vocational recovery (eg, work hardening, vocational services).
- Consultation with a pain management specialist (http://app.leg.wa.gov/wac/default.aspx?cite=246-919-863) if the worker's dose is greater than 120 mg/d MED and there is no CMIF. An electronic opioid calculator can be downloaded at http://www.agencymeddirectors.wa.gov/opioiddosing.asp. Additional appropriate consultations are recommended if the worker has a comorbid substance use or poorly controlled mental health disorder.
- Worker has no contraindication to the use of opioids.
- No evidence or likelihood of having serious adverse outcomes from opioid use.

During the chronic phase, providers should routinely review the effects of opioid therapy on function to determine whether opioid therapy should continue. COT focused only on reducing pain intensity can lead to rapidly escalating dosage with deterioration in function and quality of life. Prescribers should also continue to check the PMP and administer UDTs based on risk, in accordance with AMDG recommendations and Department of Health regulations. Because COT is associated with substantial risk for harm, opioid prescribing or dose increases that do not result in CMIF is considered not proper and necessary in the Washington State workers' compensation system.

Continued coverage of COT will depend on the prescriber documenting the following:

- CMIF is maintained, or pain interference with function score is 4 or less with stable dosing. If COT dose is increased, CMIF must be demonstrated in response to the dose change.
- A current treatment agreement is signed.
- The worker has no relative contraindication to the use of opioids.
- There is no evidence of serious adverse outcomes from opioid use.
- There has been consultation with a pain management specialist if the worker's dose is greater than 120 mg/d MED and there is no CMIF. An electronic opioid calculator can be downloaded at http://www.agencymeddirectors.wa.gov/opioiddosing.asp. Additional appropriate consultations are recommended if the worker has a comorbid substance use or poorly controlled mental health disorder.
- No aberrant behavior is identified by PMP or UDT.

Prescribers should discontinue opioids if all the above criteria are not met. Please see later discussion of Discontinuing COT.

Opioids for Catastrophic Injuries

Catastrophic injuries, such as severe burns, crush, or spinal cord injury in which significant recovery of physical function is not expected, are exempt from the above coverage criteria. For catastrophic injuries, continued use of COT may be appropriate when the prescriber has documented the following:

- A current signed treatment agreement.
- Stable opioid dose at or less than 120 mg/d MED.
- When opioid dose is greater than 120 mg/d MED, a consultation with a pain specialist is documented before further dose escalation. An electronic opioid calculator can be downloaded at http://www.agencymeddirectors.wa.gov/opioiddosing.asp.
- Worker has no relative contraindication to the use of opioids.
- No evidence of serious adverse outcomes from opioid use.
- No aberrant behavior identified by PMP or UDT.

MANAGING SURGICAL PAIN IN WORKERS ON CHRONIC OPIOID THERAPY

Managing pain in workers on COT who are undergoing elective surgeries presents unique challenges and requires a coordinated treatment plan for pain management before surgery. This coordinated treatment plan requires a collaborative effort involving the surgeon, anesthesiologist, pain management specialist, attending provider (AP), and the worker.

In general, patients on COT will report higher pain scores and manifest more anxiety than other patients.[32,33] They will also likely require higher opioid doses in the intraoperative and postoperative period. COT patients undergoing surgery have more frequent and more deadly respiratory depressive episodes than opioid-naive patients.[32]

Based on the lack of evidence, there is no consensus on whether to taper chronic opioids before elective surgery.

A preoperative evaluation is recommended, preferably by an anesthesiologist, 1 to 2 weeks before surgery. This evaluation should include the worker's current opioid dose (both prescribed and actually taken) and a thorough medical history that includes mental health and substance use disorder information. Accurate dosage information is especially important for planning perioperative pain management, yet only 9% of patients taking opioids preoperatively have dosage information in the chart.[32] The evaluator should also check the opioid prescribing history in the PMP. The following recommendations will help manage the workers' pain and minimize their risk associated with surgery.

Before surgery (preoperatively), the surgeon and AP should:

- Have a coordinated treatment plan for managing surgical pain, including identifying the postoperative opioid prescriber.
- Obtain a preoperative anesthesia consult, as above. Workers on buprenorphine need special anesthesia care and should have a consult at least 2 weeks before surgery.
- Access the PMP and review the worker's controlled substance history to get accurate information on opioid dose and concurrent medication use. Provider should discuss any apparent discrepancies with the worker.
- Prepare the worker for elective surgery by setting appropriate expectations for pain management. Workers need reassurance that their pain management needs

will be met, and they need to know that their opioid use is expected to return to the preoperative dose, or less, following surgery.

- Consider an opioid taper, but this is not required. Avoid escalating opioid dose before surgery.
- Avoid prescribing new benzodiazepines or sedative-hypnotics.
- Consider a consult with a pain management specialist before surgery for workers on high-dose opioids or who have comorbid mental health or substance use disorder.

Day of surgery (intraoperatively), the anesthesiologist should:

- Use anti-inflammatories, acetaminophen, or both, if not contraindicated.
- Continue preoperative opioids to decrease the risk of withdrawal symptoms and use regional blocks, if appropriate.
- Consider the use of other nonopioid analgesic adjuncts (eg, gabapentin, ketamine, or lidocaine) for opioid-sparing effects.

After surgery (postoperatively), the surgeon or hospitalist and AP should:

- Continue preoperative opioids, with extra analgesia for acute pain via patient-controlled analgesia (PCA) while hospitalized.
- Use care when transitioning from PCA to oral opioids. DO NOT perform a "straight" conversion from intravenous to oral opioid because of a lack of complete cross-tolerance.
- Expect the worker to need more time than other patients to stabilize pain control after transitioning to oral opioids.
- Discharge the worker on the same preoperative opioid regimen and only supplement with short-acting (not extended-release) opioids for postoperative pain.
- Do not prescribe long-acting or extended-release opioids for postoperative pain unless the worker was previously maintained on these drugs.
- Avoid new sedative-hypnotics and benzodiazepines.
- Taper total opioids to preoperative dose or lower by 6 weeks.
- Consult a specialist for workers on high-dose opioids or who have comorbid mental health or substance use disorder, if needed.

DISCONTINUING CHRONIC OPIOID THERAPY

Safety and efficacy of long-term opioid use, particularly in the injured worker population, have not been established. Discontinuation of opioids (**Box 2**) frequently improves function and quality of life and usually does not lead to increased pain levels.[34] In most cases, it is best to taper opioids off completely.

Step 1: Discontinuing Opioids in a Community Care Setting

In most cases, workers who are not on chronic high-dose opioids or who do not have comorbid substance use disorder or a significant mental health disorder may be tapered in a straightforward manner. A gradual taper of approximately 10% per week (see AMDG Guideline, Tapering or Discontinuing Opioids and Appendix H) can be carried out by the AP. Adjuvant agents like clonidine and psychological support such as cognitive behavioral therapy can be provided to assist with the taper process. The AP may also seek consultative assistance from a pain management specialist.

Box 2
Case definition: When to discontinue chronic opioid therapy

- Worker or AP requests opioid taper, OR

- Worker is maintained on opioids for at least 3 months and there is no sustained CMIF, as measured by validated instruments, OR

- Worker's risk from continued treatment outweighs benefit, OR

- Worker has experienced a severe adverse outcome or overdose event, OR

- Evidence of aberrant behavior (inconsistent UDT result, lost prescriptions, multiple requests for early refills, multiple prescribers, unauthorized dose escalation, apparent intoxication), OR

- Use of opioids is not consistent with AMDG Guideline or this guideline. In addition, medical boards in several states have recently updated their pain rules or guidelines.

  o WA: http://www.doh.wa.gov/ForPublicHealthandHealthcareProviders/HealthcareProfessions andFacilities/PainManagement/AdoptedRules;

  o NM: http://www.nmmb.state.nm.us/pdffiles/Rules/NMAC16.10.14_PainManagement.pdf;

  o OH: http://www.med.ohio.gov/pdf/NEWS/Prescribing%20Opioids%20Guidlines.pdf

  o IN: http://www.in.gov/pla/files/Emergency_Rules_Adopted_10.24.2013.pdf;

  o CA: http://www.mbc.ca.gov/About_Us/Meetings/2014/Materials/materials_20140929_rx-2.pdf;

  o CO: http://cdn.colorado.gov/cs/Satellite?blobcol=urldata&blobheadername1=Content-Disposition&blobheadername2=Content-Type&blobheadervalue1=inline%3B+filename %3D%22Opioid+Policy+Revised+10.15.14.pdf%22&blobheadervalue2=application%2F pdf&blobkey=id&blobtable=MungoBlobs&blobwhere=1252043147327&ssbinary=true

---

Step 2: Discontinuing Opioids in an Intensive Setting

For those workers who have failed step 1 or who are at high risk for failure due to high-dose, concurrent benzodiazepine use, or comorbid substance use or mental health disorder, the prescriber should consider seeking consultative assistance from a pain management specialist, a structured intensive multidisciplinary program (SIMP) provider, or addiction medicine specialist. Adjuvant agents and psychological support can be provided to assist with the taper process. In these situations, formal inpatient detoxification or a 4-week SIMP treatment program may be required.

Because of the lack of high-quality evidence of safety and comparative efficacy, ultrarapid detoxification (eg, within 3 days), using antagonist drugs with or without sedation, is not recommended.

Additional Services

If a worker has failed steps 1 and 2 AND meets the DSM-5 criteria for opioid use disorder, referral for addiction treatment through a licensed chemical dependency treatment center should be considered. There are several treatment options available for opioid use disorder. A combination of medication and behavioral therapies has been found to be most successful (Substance Abuse and Mental Health Services Administration Medication-Assisted Treatment for Opioid Addiction in Opioid Treatment Program www.kap.samhsa.gov/products/trainingcurriculums/pdfs/tip43_curriculum.pdf).

Treatment Options for Opioid Use Disorder
• Medication-assisted treatment
○ Buprenorphine (Subutex, Suboxone)
○ Methadone
○ Naltrexone (Depade, Revia, Vivitrol)
• Drug-free outpatient treatment
• Residential treatment

SUMMARY

Over the past decade, there has been a dramatic increase in the use of opioids to treat chronic noncancer pain. Opioids are also being prescribed in stronger potencies and larger doses for musculoskeletal injuries. In some cases, the use of opioids for work-related injuries may actually increase the likelihood of disability. Chronic use of opioids is strongly associated with the occurrence of dependence, particularly in the presence of comorbid mental health conditions. In addition to the risk of mortality, COT is associated with significant risk of nonfatal adverse outcomes. Because of all these potential risks, this guideline focuses on carefully assessing the risks and benefits of prescribing opioids for injured workers, particularly if they are being considered for chronic (>3 months) use. In addition, this guideline provides guidance on perioperative use of opioids, an algorithm for tapering COT, and a clear definition of meaningful improvement in function.

REFERENCES

1. Centers for Disease Control and Prevention (CDC). Increase in poisoning deaths caused by non-illicit drugs–Utah, 1991-2003. MMWR Morb Mortal Wkly Rep 2005;54(2):33–6.
2. Franklin GM, Mai J, Wickizer T, et al. Opioid dosing trends and mortality in Washington State workers' compensation, 1996-2002. Am J Ind Med 2005;48(2):91–9.
3. Paulozzi LJ, Budnitz DS, Xi Y. Increasing deaths from opioid analgesics in the United States. Pharmacoepidemiol Drug Saf 2006;15(9):618–27.
4. Centers for Disease Control and Prevention (CDC). CDC grand rounds: prescription drug overdoses—a U.S. epidemic. MMWR Morb Mortal Wkly Rep 2012; 61(1):10–3.
5. Dembe A, Wickizer T, Sieck C, et al. Opioid use and dosing in the workers' compensation setting. A comparative review and new data from Ohio. Am J Ind Med 2012;55(4):313–24.
6. Franklin GM, Rahman EA, Turner JA, et al. Opioid use for chronic low back pain: a prospective, population-based study among injured workers in Washington state, 2002-2005. Clin J Pain 2009;25(9):743–51.
7. Swedlow A, Ireland J, Johnson G. Prescribing patterns of schedule II opioids in California workers' compensation. 2011. Available at: http://www.cwci.org/research.html. Accessed May 15, 2015.
8. Washington Agency Medical Directors' Group. Interagency guideline on opioid dosing for chronic non-cancer pain: an educational pilot to improve care and safety with opioid treatment. Available at: http://www.agencymeddirectors.wa.gov/opioiddosing.asp. Accessed May 15, 2015.

9. Franklin GM, Mai J, Turner J, et al. Bending the prescription opioid dosing and mortality curves: impact of the Washington State opioid dosing guideline. Am J Ind Med 2012;55(4):325–31.

10. Franklin GM, Stover BD, Turner JA, et al. Early opioid prescription and subsequent disability among workers with back injuries: the disability risk identification study cohort. Spine (Phila Pa 1976) 2008;33(2):199–204.

11. Bernacki EJ, Yuspeh L, Lavin R, et al. Increases in the use and cost of opioids to treat acute and chronic pain in injured workers, 1999 to 2009. J Occup Environ Med 2012;54(2):216–23.

12. White JA, Tao X, Talreja M, et al. The effect of opioid use on workers' compensation claim cost in the State of Michigan. J Occup Environ Med 2012;54(8): 948–53.

13. Chou R, Qaseem A, Snow V, et al. Diagnosis and treatment of low back pain: a joint clinical practice guideline from the American College of Physicians and the American Pain Society. Ann Intern Med 2007;147(7):478–91.

14. van Tulder M, Becker A, Bekkering T, et al. Chapter 3. European guidelines for the management of acute nonspecific low back pain in primary care. Eur Spine J 2006;15(Suppl 2):S169–91.

15. Dunn KM, Saunders KW, Rutter CM, et al. Opioid prescriptions for chronic pain and overdose: a cohort study. Ann Intern Med 2010;152(2):85–92.

16. Bohnert AS, Valenstein M, Bair MJ, et al. Association between opioid prescribing patterns and opioid overdose-related deaths. JAMA 2011;305(13):1315–21.

17. Gomes T, Mamdani MM, Dhalla IA, et al. Opioid dose and drug-related mortality in patients with nonmalignant pain. Arch Intern Med 2011;171(7):686–91.

18. Chang G, Chen L, Mao J. Opioid tolerance and hyperalgesia. Med Clin North Am 2007;91(2):199–211.

19. Von Korff M, Ormel J, Keefe FJ, et al. Grading the severity of chronic pain. Pain 1992;50(2):133–49.

20. Dworkin RH, Turk DC, Wyrwich KW, et al. Interpreting the clinical importance of treatment outcomes in chronic pain clinical trials: IMMPACT recommendations. J Pain 2008;9(2):105–21.

21. Ostelo RW, Deyo RA, Stratford P, et al. Interpreting change scores for pain and functional status in low back pain: towards international consensus regarding minimal important change. Spine (Phila Pa 1976) 2008;33(1):90–4.

22. Quality of Life Scale. The American Chronic Pain Association. Available at: http://theacpa.org/uploads/documents/Life_Scale_3.pdf. Accessed May 15, 2015.

23. Edlund MJ, Martin BC, Devries A, et al. Trends in use of opioids for chronic non-cancer pain among individuals with mental health and substance use disorders: the TROUP study. Clin J Pain 2010;26(1):1–8.

24. Edlund MJ, Steffick D, Hudson T, et al. Risk factors for clinically recognized opioid abuse and dependence among veterans using opioids for chronic non-cancer pain. Pain 2007;129(3):355–62.

25. Sullivan MD, Edlund MJ, Zhang L, et al. Association between mental health disorders, problem drug use, and regular prescription opioid use. Arch Intern Med 2006;166(19):2087–93.

26. Cicero TJ, Wong G, Tian Y, et al. Co-morbidity and utilization of medical services by pain patients receiving opioid medications: data from an insurance claims database. Pain 2009;144(1–2):20–7.

27. Skurtveit S, Furu K, Selmer R, et al. Nicotine dependence predicts repeated use of prescribed opioids. Prospective population-based cohort study. Ann Epidemiol 2010;20(12):890–7.

28. Braden JB, Sullivan MD, Ray GT, et al. Trends in long-term opioid therapy for non-cancer pain among persons with a history of depression. Gen Hosp Psychiatry 2009;31(6):564–70.
29. Saunders KW, Dunn KM, Merrill JO, et al. Relationship of opioid use and dosage levels to fractures in older chronic pain patients. J Gen Intern Med 2010;25(4):310–5.
30. Martin BC, Fan MY, Edlund MJ, et al. Long-term chronic opioid therapy discontinuation rates from the TROUP study. J Gen Intern Med 2011;26(12):1450–7.
31. Chou R, Fanciullo GJ, Fine PG, et al. Clinical guidelines for the use of chronic opioid therapy in chronic noncancer pain. J Pain 2009;10(2):113–30.
32. Rapp SE, Ready LB, Nessly ML. Acute pain management in patients with prior opioid consumption: a case-controlled retrospective review. Pain 1995;61(2):195–201.
33. Theunissen M, Peters ML, Bruce J, et al. Preoperative anxiety and catastrophizing: a systematic review and meta-analysis of the association with chronic post-surgical pain. Clin J Pain 2012;28:819–41.
34. Jensen MP, Turner JA, Romano JM. Changes in beliefs, catastrophizing, and coping are associated with improvement in multidisciplinary pain treatment. J Consult Clin Psychol 2001;69(4):655–62.

FURTHER READING

Favrat B, Zimmermann G, Zullino D, et al. Opioid antagonist detoxification under anaesthesia versus traditional clonidine detoxification combined with an additional week of psychosocial support: a randomised clinical trial. Drug Alcohol Depend 2006;81(2):109–16.
Gandhi DH, Jaffe JH, McNary S, et al. Short-term outcomes after brief ambulatory opioid detoxification with buprenorphine in young heroin users. Addiction 2003;98(4):453–62.
Gowing L, Ali R, White JM. Opioid antagonists under heavy sedation or anaesthesia for opioid withdrawal. Cochrane Database Syst Rev 2010;(1):CD002022.
Hensel M, Kox WJ. Safety, efficacy, and long-term results of a modified version of rapid opiate detoxification under general anaesthesia: a prospective study in methadone, heroin, codeine and morphine addicts. Acta Anaesthesiol Scand 2000;44(3):326–33.
Katz EC, Schwartz RP, King S, et al. Brief vs. extended buprenorphine detoxification in a community treatment program: engagement and short-term outcomes. Am J Drug Alcohol Abuse 2009;35(2):63–7.
Krabbe PF, Koning JP, Heinen N, et al. Rapid detoxification from opioid dependence under general anaesthesia versus standard methadone tapering: abstinence rates and withdrawal distress experiences. Addict Biol 2003;8(3):351–8.
Ling W, Hillhouse M, Domier C, et al. Buprenorphine tapering schedule and illicit opioid use. Addiction 2009;104(2):256–65.
Woody GE, Poole SA, Subramaniam G, et al. Extended vs short-term buprenorphine-naloxone for treatment of opioid-addicted youth: a randomized trial. JAMA 2008;300(17):2003–11.

Shoulder Conditions
Diagnosis and Treatment Guideline

Michael Codsi, MD[a], Chris R. Howe, MD[b],*

KEYWORDS

- Shoulder guideline • Rotator cuff tear • Workers compensation

KEY POINTS

- Degenerative conditions of the shoulder and rotator cuff have a high prevalence with aging.
- Acute traumatic rotator cuff tears likely benefit from surgical intervention.
- The routine use of a distal claviculectomy during rotator cuff repair is discouraged.
- The use of allografts and xenografts in rotator cuff tear repair is not encouraged.

INTRODUCTION

This guideline is intended as an educational resource for health care providers who treat shoulder conditions, particularly injured workers. The emphasis is on accurate diagnosis and treatment that is curative or rehabilitative. The goal is to provide standards that ensure a uniform high quality of care based on the best available clinical and scientific evidence from a systematic review of the literature and on a consensus of expert opinion when scientific evidence was insufficient.

Degenerative conditions and injuries are common in both the workers' compensation and general populations. Accurate assessment and treatment are critical to ascertaining work-relatedness and facilitating the worker's return to health and productivity.

ESTABLISHING WORK-RELATEDNESS

Shoulder conditions are a common cause of pain and disability among adults, with a prevalence of 7% to 10%[1]. A shoulder condition may arise from acute trauma or, in some circumstances, from nontraumatic industrial activities.

No disclosures.
[a] EvergreeenHealth Medical Center, 12040 NE 128th st, Kirklnad, WA 98034, USA; [b] Proliance Orthopedic Associates, 4011 Talbot Road South, Suite #300, Renton, WA 98055, USA
* Corresponding author.
E-mail address: c.howe@proliancesurgeons.com

Phys Med Rehabil Clin N Am 26 (2015) 467–489
http://dx.doi.org/10.1016/j.pmr.2015.04.007
1047-9651/15/$ – see front matter © 2015 Elsevier Inc. All rights reserved.

Risk factors associated with shoulder conditions include trauma, overuse, inflammation, age-related tissue degeneration, and smoking.[2] A careful history is needed both for elucidating the mechanism of injury and for establishing causation.

Shoulder Conditions as Industrial Injuries

A shoulder condition may be induced acutely (eg, a patient falls on an outstretched hand and experiences concomitant trauma). To establish a diagnosis of a shoulder condition as a work-related injury, the provider must give a clear description of the traumatic event leading to the injury (**Table 1**).

Shoulder Conditions as Occupational Diseases

Work-related activities may cause or contribute to the development of shoulder conditions caused by chronic exposures. Conditions that support work-relatedness are

1. Carrying/lifting heavy loads on or above the shoulders or carrying with hands
2. Pushing/pulling heavy loads
3. Working with arms above the shoulder for more than 15 minutes at intervals
4. Repetitive arm/wrist movements combined with force for long periods

To establish a diagnosis of an occupational disease, all of the following *are required*:

1. Exposure: Workplace activities that contribute to or cause shoulder conditions
2. Outcome: A diagnosis of a shoulder condition that meets the diagnostic criteria in this guideline
3. Relationship: Generally accepted scientific evidence, which establishes on a more-probable-than-not basis (greater than 50%) that the workplace activities (exposure) in an individual case contributed to the development or worsening of the condition relative to the risks in everyday life; translates to an odds ratio of 2 or greater in epidemiologic studies

In order for a shoulder condition to be allowed as an occupational disease, the provider must document that the work exposures created a risk of contracting or worsening the condition relative to the risks in everyday life, on a

Table 1
Exposure and risk

Exposure	Examples of Types of Jobs	Risk	Type of Shoulder Claim
Sudden trauma or fall on an outstretched arm	Construction workers, logging, painters	High	Injury
Chronic overuse with high force and repetitive overhead motion	Shipyard welders and plate workers, fish processing workers, machine operators, ground workers (eg, pushing a lawn mower), and carpenters	Medium	Injury or occupational disease
Moderate lifting	Grocery checkers	Low	Injury or occupational disease

There is no substantial scientific evidence to support the existence of overuse syndrome (ie, an injury to one extremity causing the contralateral extremity to be damaged by overuse).

more-probable-than-not basis (*Dennis v Department of Labor and Industries*, 109WN.2d 467 (Washington 1987)).

MAKING THE DIAGNOSIS

A case definition for a shoulder condition includes appropriate symptoms, objective physical findings, and abnormal imaging. A presumptive diagnosis may be based on symptoms and objective findings, but the diagnosis usually requires confirmation by clinical imaging before proceeding to surgery.

History and Clinical Examination

A thorough occupational history is essential for determining whether a shoulder condition is work related and whether it is caused by an acute or chronic exposure. The provider should take extra care in documenting the reasons for diagnosing an occupational disease, as multiple employers might share liability. Providers should document the exposure and submit a complete work history as soon as a diagnosis of occupational disease is made (see Establishing work-relatedness).

The most typical symptom that patients with shoulder pathology describe is pain in and around the shoulder. The pain can be localized to a specific area of the shoulder, such as the anterior acromion, acromioclavicular (AC) joint, biceps groove, posterior joint line, lateral acromion, or over the middle of the deltoid several centimeters distal to the acromion. The pain can also radiate down the arm to the elbow or up the trapezius muscle to the base of the neck. Patients can also complain of intermittent tingling down the arm to the fingers. Some patients can complain of popping and grinding in the shoulder during movement. Movement of the shoulder usually makes the pain worse, and rest alleviates the pain. Some patients may have a constant ache in the shoulder that does not go away or worsens when they try to sleep at night.

Patients usually complain of decreased shoulder function because they are unable to do simple activities of daily living, such as sleeping, combing their hair, getting dressed, putting on a coat, reaching out a car window, or emptying the dishwasher. Other patients may complain of weakness in the shoulder, loss of shoulder motion, or inability to play their usual sport or hobby. For patients with work-related injuries, the most common complaint is the inability to perform their regular job duties, such as lifting overhead, pushing heavy objects, or performing repetitive activities with the arm.

Physical examination should consist of accepted test and examination techniques that should help the clinician narrow down the differential diagnosis that was made after taking the patients' history. The examination should include the neck and the elbow because the joint above or below the affected area can sometimes be the primary cause of patients' shoulder pain. The clinician should measure active range of motion; if it is not normal, then passive range of motion should also be performed. The clinician should palpate the shoulder for areas of tenderness over the acromion; AC joint; biceps groove; greater tuberosity; anterior, lateral, and posterior deltoid; posterior joint line; trapezius; and scapula. An inspection of the shoulder should be done to find any muscle atrophy, bone deformity, prior surgical scars, skin abnormalities, and dyskinesias during active shoulder movement. Specific clinical examination tests should also be done, such as the Neer impingement sign, lag sign, and so forth. More detailed descriptions of these tests can be found in Appendix.

Diagnostic Imaging

Conventional radiograph, MRI, and ultrasound are the best imaging tools to corroborate the diagnosis of a shoulder condition.[3–7] MRI has been considered the gold standard; however, research has demonstrated the efficacy of ultrasound, done by a skilled provider or technician, to diagnose rotator cuff tears. A systematic review found ultrasound to have a pooled sensitivity of 0.95 and specificity of 0.96 in detecting full-thickness rotator cuff tears.[3] Ultrasound was nearly as effective as MRI in diagnosing partial tears; therefore, ultrasound may be recommended to diagnose full- and partial-thickness tears.[5]

Contrast MRI is not necessary to diagnose rotator cuff tears but may be considered when there is suspicion of an superior labral anterior-posterior (SLAP) lesion/tear.[8,9]

TREATMENT
Conservative Treatment

Shoulder injuries may be complex, often involving more than a single tissue or anatomic element. Different shoulder problems can present with similar findings, such as limited, painful motion and tenderness. It is important to consider which components of the shoulder girdle may be affected and tailor a conservative treatment plan accordingly. Published reports have reported utility for a variety of conservative interventions to reduce pain and improve function for several shoulder conditions. However, well-designed research studies on conservative care for musculoskeletal injuries are limited in both quantity and quality.

The following is an example of a conservative intervention treatment algorithm:

- Nonsteroidal antiinflammatory drugs (NSAIDs) and acetaminophen may be considered to treat pain.[10]
- Include brief rest and immobilization (less than 4 days) in the early stage; however, early unloaded movement and manual interventions, such as mobilization and manipulation, have been reported to reduce symptoms and facilitate greater shoulder motion, especially with AC injuries.[11]
- Immobilization carries the risk of a frozen shoulder and is, therefore, not recommended, with the exception of fractures or glenohumeral dislocations.
- Use therapeutic exercise and mobilization to improve shoulder range of motion and strength and decrease pain in soft tissue injuries, such as shoulder sprain, rotator cuff tendonitis or tears, and glenohumeral dislocations.[12–14]
- Incorporate strengthening exercise once range of motion is increased and pain is reduced.[14]
- Corticosteroid injections, typically within the subacromial space, have been reported to provide short-term relief for adhesive capsulitis, rotator cuff tendinopathy, impingement syndrome, tendon disorders, and SLAP disorders.[15–18] Care must be exercised when giving a corticosteroid injection to a partial rotator cuff tear, as this may lead to tear extension. Because corticosteroid use is associated with side effects, such as weakening of connective tissue, no more than 3 injections are recommended under one claim for the shoulder, 4 injections per lifetime.
- Ergonomic interventions, such as workstation and/or work flow modification, seem to be helpful in sustaining return to work.[19–21]

Any worker who does not gain meaningful functional improvement (30%–50%) within 4 to 6 weeks of conservative treatment should be considered for a specialist consultation. Meaningful functional improvement may best be determined using validated shoulder/arm function instruments, such as the Simple Shoulder Test (SST),[22] the Shoulder Pain and Disability Index (SPADI),[23,24] the Disabilities of the Arm, Shoulder, and Hand Score (DASH) or Quick DASH,[25–28] or the American Shoulder and Elbow Surgeons Assessment (ASES)[26] form.

SPECIFIC CONDITIONS
Rotator Cuff Tears

Rotator cuff tears can be acute or chronic in onset and will vary in tendon tear size, tendon retraction, muscle atrophy, and tendon loss.

As industrial injury
A worker presenting with acute pain suspicious for a rotator cuff tear should be able to report a precipitating traumatic event, such as a severe fall on an outstretched arm, an episode of heavy lifting, or forceful use of the arm.

As occupational disease
Chronic exposure risk factors for rotator cuff tears include heavy repetitive overhead work, such as in the examples in **Table 1**. However, many rotator cuff tears are caused by non–work-related conditions, such as age-related degeneration. The likelihood of having a rotator cuff tear increases with age. Studies show that more than half of individuals aged 60 years and older have partial or complete tears, yet are asymptomatic and have no history of trauma.[29] Smoking has also been associated with rotator cuff tears.[30]

Diagnosis and treatment
A careful occupational history and good clinical examination are most important in making a diagnosis of a rotator cuff tear and relating it to work exposures. Nonspecific symptoms reported with rotator cuff tears are pain with movement and pain at night. Objective clinical findings include weakness on testing forward elevation or external rotation. Patients with a positive drop arm sign, positive painful arc, and weakness with external rotation have a 91% chance of having a rotator cuff tear based on one study.[31]

Ultrasound and conventional MRI are the best imaging tools for diagnosing rotator cuff tears.[5,7] MRI remains the gold standard in the radiographic assessment of rotator cuff tears.[32] Radiograph or computed tomography arthrogram is appropriate if there is a contraindication to an MRI. Contrast MRI is not necessary for making the diagnosis of a rotator cuff tear. Arthroscopy for the purpose of diagnosing rotator cuff tears is not appropriate.

Acute, symptomatic, full-thickness rotator cuff tears, especially in a young worker, should be surgically repaired as soon as possible because of an increased risk of tear progression, retraction of the tendon, and irreversible fatty infiltration of the rotator cuff muscles.[33] For a rotator cuff tear that was previously treated conservatively, worsening pain usually indicates tear progression or migration of the humeral head[34–36] and could warrant operative care. Tears that are found incidentally and are asymptomatic are generally not work related and can get better with conservative care.

Partial tears and chronic full-thickness tears in individuals greater than 65 years old should be treated conservatively before surgery is considered.[2] Many workers, regardless of age, can recover function without surgery.

Injured workers with full- or partial-thickness tears may continue to work with restricted use of the involved extremity, if work accommodation is allowed.

Rotator cuff repairs are increasingly done arthroscopically. Evidence does not support a difference in outcomes according to surgical technique, whether it is arthroscopic, mini-open, or single- or double-row techniques.[37] Acromioplasty is not usually necessary during a rotator cuff repair; acromioplasty does not change functional outcome after arthroscopic repair of the rotator cuff.[38–41]

Tissue grafts (ie, acellular human dermal matrix)
The use of xenografts and allografts is currently not covered, given clinical concerns about localized reactions and a lack of studies demonstrating superiority to conventional techniques. There is an increased risk of infection and rejection reported with the use of xenografts, and there is no difference in outcome when they are used.[42]

Distal clavicle resection as a routine part of acute rotator cuff tear repair is not recommended.

Revision rotator cuff repairs

Nicotine has been associated with delayed tendon-to-bone healing after rotator cuff tear repair surgery.[30,43–45] It is strongly recommended that revision surgery not be performed in current nicotine users. Revision rotator cuff surgery should not be done if a patient has a massive rotator cuff tear (ie, tears >3 cm or with severe fatty infiltration). The outcome of revision surgery for symptomatic failed primary repairs is inferior to a successful primary repair.[46]

A second revision surgery or subsequent surgeries will only be considered if compelling evidence exists that the injured worker had returned to a state of clinically meaningful functional improvement (at least 30%) after the last revision surgery, followed by an ongoing significant decline in function. Measures of functional improvement should be documented on a validated instrument (eg, DASH, SST, SPADI, and ASES) for a second revision surgery to be allowed.

Subacromial Impingement Syndrome Without a Rotator Cuff Tear

Subacromial impingement syndrome (SIS) results when the soft tissues of the shoulder between the coracoacromial arch and the humeral tuberosity are compressed, disturbing the normal sliding mechanism of the shoulder when the arm is elevated. Inflammation of the subacromial bursa, tendinopathy of the rotator cuff tendons, and acromial morphology can all contribute to the development of SIS. SIS can be an occupational disease; it has been associated with heavy overhead work, high force, and repetition of shoulder movement.[47]

Diagnosis and treatment

Workers may report generalized shoulder pain. An objective clinical finding is pain over the anterior or lateral shoulder during active elevation as well as a positive Neer or Hawkins impingement sign. To confirm the diagnosis of SIS, a radiograph should reveal abnormal acromion morphology with narrowing of the subacromial space or an MRI should reveal evidence of tendinopathy/tendinitis of the rotator cuff tendon or fluid or inflammation in the subacromial bursa.

Nonoperative treatments of SIS have been shown to be as effective as subacromial decompression.[48,49] For decompression to be allowed for SIS, the diagnosis must be verified by pain relief from a subacromial injection of local anesthetic and the worker must have failed to improve function and decrease pain after 12 weeks of conservative care.

Subacromial decompression is also a reasonable treatment option for massive, irreparable rotator cuff tears that are not amenable to repair and have not improved with a course of physical therapy.

Calcific Tendonitis

The exact cause of calcific tendonitis is still unknown. It does, however, affect up to 10% to 20% of the population between 30 and 50 years of age.[50–52]

Diagnosis and treatment

The diagnosis of calcific tendonitis is typically made with conventional plain films alone. Calcific tendonitis is not always symptomatic. When calcific tendonitis is symptomatic, nonoperative treatment of the condition is typically successful.[50,53] If symptoms continue after 12 weeks of conservative management, then debridement of the calcified tendon is reasonable.

Acromioclavicular Dislocation

Acute AC injury is typically referred to as shoulder separation. The degree of clavicular displacement depends on the severity of the injury. The injury is classified using the Rockwood classification[54] (**Table 2**).

Diagnosis and treatment

AC dislocations (types III-VI) show marked deformity and are accompanied by pain and tenderness over the AC joint. Conventional radiograph is the best imaging tool to use when AC dislocation is suspected.

Surgery is not covered for type I and II injuries, whereas surgery is usually indicated for types IV, V, and VI. Management of type III injuries is more controversial but most patients with type III AC joint dislocations are best treated conservatively. Surgery should be considered only when at least 3 months of conservative care fails. For patients with a type III dislocation and high physical demands on the shoulder, early orthopedic surgical consultation and/or surgery may be indicated.

Labral Tears, Including Superior Labral Anterior-Posterior Tears

Labral lesions constitute a wide range of pathology. The most common labral lesions are SLAP tears (**Table 3**), which are superior labral tears that extend anteriorly and posteriorly. Some SLAP tears result from acute trauma and others are degenerative

Table 2 Rockwood classification of AC injuries	
Rockwood Classification	
Type I	There is sprain of the AC or coracoclavicular ligament.
Type II	Subluxation of the AC joint is associated with a tear of the AC ligament; coracoclavicular ligament is intact.
Type III	There is dislocation of the AC joint with injury to both AC and coracoclavicular ligaments.
Type IV	Clavicle is displaced posteriorly through the trapezius muscle.
Type V	There is gross disparity between the acromion and clavicle, which displaces superiorly.
Type VI	Dislocated lateral end of the clavicle lies inferior to the coracoid.

Types I to III are common, whereas types IV to VI are rare.

Table 3	
Types of SLAP tears	
Tear Type	Description
I	There is fraying of the labrum without detachment from the glenoid.
II	The labrum is completely torn off the glenoid. Type II SLAP tears are subdivided into a. Anterior b. Posterior c. Combined anterior and posterior
III	Bucket handle tear: The torn labrum hangs into the joint and causes symptoms of "locking, popping."
IV	Labral tear extends into the long head of the biceps tendon.

in nature. There are several types of SLAP tears; type II SLAP tears are the most common and constitute more than 50% of all tears.[55,56]

Diagnosis and treatment

No single examination technique is highly specific or sensitive in diagnosing labral tears because patients often have concomitant pathology. Some signs and symptoms include locking, popping, and grinding sensation, and pain worse when doing activities[57] Physical examination (eg, the O'Brien test, Speed test, Yergason test, or other labral loading test) must be positive in addition to finding a labral tear on imaging to confirm the diagnosis. Conventional MRI may be used, but MRI with contrast has the highest reported sensitivity and specificity for the diagnosis of SLAP tears.[8,58–61]

Because most SLAP tears are associated with other pathology, the provider should identify other shoulder conditions, if any, and follow appropriate surgical indications. Operative treatment of labral tears depends on the type of tear that is present and may include debridement, repair of the labrum, or biceps tenodesis depending on the type of tear found at the time of surgery.[62–66] Literature suggests that there are no advantages to repairing type II lesions associated with rotator cuff tears in patients older than 50 years of age.[64] Indications for surgery for SLAP tears are not standardized and remain somewhat controversial. Expert opinion, including the American Academy of Orthopedic Surgeons, recommends initial conservative care management for SLAP tears. In general, conservative care management should last a minimum of 6 to 12 weeks. Early surgery should be considered only in cases when there is evidence of symptomatic suprascapular nerve compression by an associated paralabral cyst that was caused by a labral tear.

Acromioclavicular Arthritis

AC arthritis may result from previous trauma to the joint or may be the result of heavy lifting over a period of time.

Diagnosis and treatment

Symptoms include pain and tenderness at the AC joint. Symptomatic AC arthritis may initially improve with steroid injection. During rotator cuff repair, the decision to resect the distal clavicle should be based on radiograph, MRI (radiologist interpreted), or bone scan showing moderate to severe AC joint arthritis, distal clavicle edema, or distal clavicle osteolysis.

Claviculectomy/Mumford as an add-on or as a stand-alone procedure should meet all criteria (**Table 4**) and should not be done without the specified objective

Table 4
Review criteria for shoulder surgery

| A Request May be Appropriate for | If Patients Have | AND the Diagnosis is Supported by These Clinical Findings: | | | AND This has Been Done (if Recommended) |
Surgical Procedure	Diagnosis	Subjective	Objective	Imaging	Nonoperative Care
Rotator cuff tear repair Note: The use of allografts and xenografts in rotator cuff tear repair is not encouraged. Note: Distal clavicle resection as a routine part of acute rotator cuff tear repair is not covered.	Acute full-thickness rotator cuff tear	Report of an acute traumatic injury within 3 mo of seeking care AND Shoulder pain with movement and/or at night	Patients will usually have weakness with one or more of the following: • Forward elevation • Internal/external rotation • Abduction testing	Conventional radiographs, AP and true lateral or axillary view AND MRI, ultrasound, or radiographic arthrogram reveals a full-thickness rotator cuff tear Routine use of contrast imaging is not indicated	May be offered but not required
Rotator cuff tear repair	Partial-thickness rotator cuff tear	Pain with active arc motion 90°–130°	Weak or painful abduction AND Tenderness over rotator cuff AND Positive impingement sign	Conventional radiographs, AP and true lateral or axillary view AND MRI, ultrasound, or radiographic arthrogram shows a partial-thickness rotator cuff tear Routine use of contrast imaging is not indicated	Conservative care[a] required for at least 6 wk, then: If tear is >50% of the tendon thickness, may consider surgery If <50% thickness, do 6 more weeks conservative care

(continued on next page)

Table 4
(continued)

A Request May be Appropriate for	If Patients Have	AND the Diagnosis is Supported by These Clinical Findings:			AND This has Been Done (if Recommended)
Surgical Procedure	Diagnosis	Subjective	Objective	Imaging	Nonoperative Care
Rotator cuff tear repair Note: The use of allografts and xenografts in rotator cuff tear repair is not encouraged.	Chronic or degenerative full-thickness rotator cuff tear	Gradual onset of shoulder pain without a traumatic event OR Minor trauma, night pain	Patients will usually have weakness with one or more of the following: • Forward elevation • Internal/external rotation • Abduction testing	Conventional radiographs, AP and true lateral or axillary view AND MRI, ultrasound, or radiographic arthrogram reveals a full-thickness rotator cuff tear Routine use of contrast imaging is not indicated	Conservative care[a] for at least 6 wk If no improvement after 6 wk, and tear is repairable, surgery may be considered
Rotator cuff tear repair after previous rotator cuff surgery 1. One revision surgery may be considered. Revision surgery is not recommended in the presence of a massive rotator cuff tear, as defined by one or more of the following: 1. >3 cm of retraction 2. severe rotator cuff muscle atrophy 3. severe fatty infiltration	Recurring full-thickness tear	New traumatic injury with good function before injury	Patients may have weakness with forward elevation, internal/external rotation, and/or abduction testing	Conventional radiographs, AP and true lateral or axillary view AND MRI, ultrasound, or radiographic arthrogram reveals a full-thickness rotator cuff tear Routine use of contrast imaging is not indicated	Conservative care[a] for at least 6 wk If no improvement after 6 wk, and tear is repairable, surgery may be considered

2. Second and subsequent revisions Revision surgery is *not recommended* in the presence of a massive rotator cuff tear, as defined by one or more of the following: 1. >3 cm of retraction 2. Severe rotator cuff muscle atrophy 3. Severe fatty infiltration	Recurring full-thickness tear	2. No new injury but gradual onset of pain with good function for over a year after previous surgery Second revision will only be considered when patients have returned to work or have clinically meaningful improvement in function, on validated instrument, after the most recent surgery	Patients may have weakness with forward elevation, internal/external rotation, and/or abduction testing	Conventional radiographs, AP and true lateral or axillary view **AND** MRI, ultrasound, or radiographic arthrogram reveals a full-thickness rotator cuff tear Routine use of contrast imaging is not indicated	Second revision: Conservative care[a] for 6 wk is recommended; if no improvement, surgery may be considered
Partial claviculectomy (includes Mumford procedure) *Not recommended as a part of acute rotator cuff repair* *Note:* Mumford procedure done alone must meet all these criteria. Mumford as an add-on to any other shoulder surgery must also meet all diagnostic criteria preoperatively. Intraoperative visualization of AC joint, in the absence of radiographic findings, is not a	Arthritis of AC joint	Pain at AC joint; aggravation of pain with shoulder motion	Tenderness over the AC joint **AND** *Documented* pain relief with an anesthetic injection	MRI (radiologist interpretation) reveals: • Moderate to severe degenerative joint disease of AC joint, or • Distal clavicle edema, or • Osteolysis of distal clavicle **OR** Bone scan is positive **OR** Radiologist's interpretation of radiograph reveals moderate to severe AC joint arthritis	Conservative care[a] for at least 6 wk (if done in isolation) Surgery is not indicated before 6 wk

(continued on next page)

Table 4
(continued)

A Request May be Appropriate for	If Patients Have	AND the Diagnosis is Supported by These Clinical Findings:			AND This has Been Done (if Recommended)
Surgical Procedure	Diagnosis	Subjective	Objective	Imaging	Nonoperative Care
sufficient finding to authorize the claviculectomy.					
Isolated subacromial decompression with or without acromioplasty	Subacromial impingement syndrome	Generalized shoulder pain	Pain with active elevation	MRI reveals evidence of tendinopathy/ tendinitis OR A rotator cuff tear	12 wk of conservative care[a] AND Subacromial injection with local anesthetic gives documented pain relief
Debridement of calcific tendonitis	Calcific tendonitis	Generalized shoulder pain	Pain with active elevation	Conventional radiographs show calcium deposit in the rotator cuff	12 wk of conservative care[a]
Open treatment of acute AC dislocation *Note*: Surgery for acute types I and II AC joint dislocations is not recommended.	Shoulder AC joint separation	Pain with marked functional difficulty	Marked deformity	Conventional radiographs show type III or greater separation	Conservative care[a] only for types I and II Conservative care for 3 mo for type III separations, with the exception of early surgery being considered for heavy or overhead laborers Immediate surgical intervention for types IV-VI

Repair, debridement, or biceps tenodesis for labral lesion, including SLAP tears	Labral tears without instability (including SLAP tears)	Traumatic event reported or an occupation with significant overhead activity **AND** Pain worse with motion and active elevation	Pain reproduced with labral loading tests (eg, O'Brien test)	MRI shows labral tear	At least 6 wk of conservative care[a]
Capsulorrhaphy (Bankart procedure)	Glenohumeral instability	History of a dislocation that inhibits activities of daily living	Positive apprehension/ relocation test	Conventional radiographs **AND** MRI demonstrates one of the following: 1. Bankart/labral lesion 2. Hill Sachs lesion 3. Capsular tear	If only one dislocation has occurred, recommend 1–2 wk of immobilization then PT for 6–8 wk; if a positive apprehension present at 6 wk, surgery may be considered 2 or more dislocations in 3 mo may proceed to surgery without conservative care Early surgery may be considered in patients with large bone defects or in patients <35 y old
Tenodesis or tenotomy of long head of biceps	Partial biceps tear, biceps instability from the biceps groove, proximal biceps enlargement that inhibits gliding in the biceps groove, complete tear of the proximal biceps tendon	Anterior shoulder pain, weakness, and deformity	Tenderness over the biceps groove, pain in the anterior shoulder during resisted supination of the forearm Partial-thickness tears do not have the classic appearance of ruptured muscle	MRI required if procedure performed in isolation; if biceps tendon pathology identified and addressed during separate procedure, the code may be added retroactively	Surgery almost never considered in full-thickness ruptures

(continued on next page)

Table 4
(continued)

A Request May be Appropriate for	If Patients Have	AND the Diagnosis is Supported by These Clinical Findings:			AND This has Been Done (if Recommended)
Surgical Procedure	Diagnosis	Subjective	Objective	Imaging	Nonoperative Care
Total/hemi shoulder arthroplasty	Severe proximal humerus fracture with posttraumatic arthritis, posttraumatic avascular necrosis OR Comminuted fractures of proximal humerus	Pain with ROM, history of work-related fracture	Pain/crepitus with ROM, decreased ROM	Conventional radiographs show moderate to severe glenohumeral arthritis OR Avascular necrosis OR Comminuted fractures of proximal humerus	Conservative care[a] may be offered but not required
Reverse total shoulder arthroplasty	Rotator cuff arthropathy OR Severe proximal humerus fractures	Pain, weakness AND History of work-related rotator cuff tear	Inability to elevate arm, pain with ROM	Conventional radiographs show moderate to severe glenohumeral arthritis and a high-riding humeral head	Conservative care[a] may be offered but not required
Manipulation under anesthesia/ arthroscopic capsular release	Idiopathic adhesive capsulitis, postoperative adhesive capsulitis	Pain, loss of motion	Loss of passive motion	Conventional radiographs do not show bone pathology that can explain the loss of motion	12 wk of conservative care[a]
Diagnostic arthroscopy	Arthroscopy for diagnostic purposes	*Diagnostic arthroscopy is not recommended.*			

Abbreviations: AP, anteroposterior; PT, physical therapy; ROM, range of motion.
[a] Conservative care should include at least active assisted range of motion and home-based exercises.

findings. It is important to document the source of pain, including pain relief with local anesthetic injection.

The routine use of the Mumford procedure during a rotator cuff tear repair is discouraged.

Glenohumeral Dislocation

Glenohumeral dislocations typically involve a soft tissue injury, such as a rotator cuff tear or a tear of the glenohumeral ligament.

Diagnosis and treatment

The inability to move the shoulder after an acute injury, shoulder deformity, and weakness are the main symptoms. Dislocations that are not accompanied by tears can be treated by reduction of the humeral head and initial immobilization followed by structured rehabilitation.

Surgical interventions have been shown to reduce the rate of recurrent instability in young (younger than 35 years) active patients with first-time dislocation.[67,68] When a dislocation is associated with a rotator cuff tear, then repair of the tear is appropriate without additional conservative care. If the dislocation is associated with a labral tear, then initial conservative care is reasonable.

If instability persists after 6 weeks of conservative care, surgery is warranted. Surgery may also be appropriate if there is a history of more than one dislocation in a 3-month period. Arthroscopic and open labral/Bankart (capsulorraphy) repairs yield similar results in regard to recurrent instability, clinical outcomes, and postoperative osteoarthritis.[69,70] *Thermal capsulorrhaphy is not recommended,* as there is no evidence of benefit.[71]

Typically multidirectional instability is not considered a work-related injury or an occupational disease. It is an acknowledged pathologic condition seen in the normal population, but surgery is typically not indicated.

Tendon Rupture or Tendinopathy of the Long Head of the Biceps

Tendinopathy of the long head of the biceps most commonly presents in combination with rotator cuff tears, SLAP lesions, and subacromial bursitis.

Diagnosis and treatment

Patients typically present with increasing anterior shoulder pain, declining function, and a history of chronic repetitive overhead use. An MRI or an ultrasound may reveal tendinopathy, a partial tear, or a complete tear of the tendon; however, all imaging studies lack sensitivity and specificity as compared with arthroscopy.

For proximal long head biceps tendon rupture, active participation in conservative treatment is often successful; however, surgery may be indicated in young active patients. Nonsurgical management should be initiated for tendinopathy. Surgery may be considered for symptomatic partial tears and medial subluxation of the tendon. Tenotomy and tenodesis have comparable favorable results in literature, with the only major difference being a higher incidence of deformity with biceps tenotomy.[63,72] Tenodesis may be preferred for younger patients to avoid a cosmetic deformity or for patients who use the biceps for heavy lifting at work to avoid biceps cramping.[73]

Glenohumeral Arthritis and Arthropathy

Treatment of degenerative conditions, such as glenohumeral arthritis or rotator cuff tear, arthropathy is generally initiated with nonoperative management techniques, such as NSAIDs and physical therapy. Conservative management is not, however, mandatory if severe degenerative changes are noted on conventional radiographs, as the likelihood of meaningful long-term relief is negligible.

Arthroplasties are a treatment option for acute comminuted fractures, posttraumatic arthritis, glenohumeral arthritis, and rotator cuff tear arthropathy. Total shoulder arthroplasties are primarily used to treat glenohumeral arthritis. Reverse shoulder arthroplasties have become the treatment of choice for the management of rotator cuff tear arthropathy whereby the glenohumeral arthritis is associated with a chronic rotator cuff tear and a high-riding humerus.

All conditions are heralded by pain and limitations in range of motion. Conventional radiographs are typically sufficient to make the diagnosis of any of the preceding conditions.

Highly comminuted fractures of the proximal humerus may not always be repairable. If deemed irreparable, then proceeding to a hemiarthroplasty urgently or emergently is reasonable.

Manipulation Under Anesthesia/Arthroscopic Capsular Release

Manipulation under anesthesia, or arthroscopic capsular release, may be considered if a patient has persistent stiffness, typically after a procedure that has not responded to at least 12 weeks of physical therapy and/or directed home exercises.

Diagnostic Arthroscopy

Diagnostic arthroscopy is not currently accepted as a viable treatment option. If conventional radiographs and an MRI are unable to identify an anatomic explanation for a workers pain, then surgery should not be performed.

Table 5 SST		
Simply Circle Yes or No		
1. Is your shoulder comfortable with your arm at rest by your side?	Yes	No
2. Does your shoulder allow you to sleep comfortably?	Yes	No
3. Can you reach the small of your back to tuck in your shirt with your hand?	Yes	No
4. Can you place your hand behind your head with the elbow straight out to the side?	Yes	No
5. Can you place a coin on a shelf at the level of your shoulder without bending your elbow?	Yes	No
6. Can you lift 1 lb (a full pint container) to the level of your shoulder without bending your elbow?	Yes	No
7. Can you lift 8 lb (a full gallon container) to the level of the top of your head without bending your elbow?	Yes	No
8. Can you carry 20 lb (a bag of potatoes) at your side with the affected arm?	Yes	No
9. Do you think you can toss a softball underhand 10 yards with the affected arm?	Yes	No
10. Do you think you can throw a softball overhand 20 yards with the affected arm?	Yes	No
11. Can you wash the back of your opposite shoulder with the affected arm?	Yes	No
12. Would your shoulder allow you to work full time at your regular job?	Yes	No
Score (total number of No's)		

From Godfrey J, Hammoan R, Lowenstein S, et al. Reliability, validity, and responsiveness of the simple shoulder test: psychometric properties by age and injury type. J Shoulder Elbow Surg 2007;16:260–7.

POSTOPERATIVE TREATMENT AND RETURN TO WORK

It is important for the attending provider and the surgeon to focus on preoperative planning for postoperative recovery, reactivation, and return-to-work activities. During the immediate postoperative period (6 weeks), the surgeon should be involved in helping to direct these activities.

Unless a patient has multiple injuries, return to work within 6 weeks after surgery is reasonable if appropriate modifications are available.

Work accommodation during the early recovery periods with conservative interventions seems to be well supported. Jobsite modifications depend on the nature of the

Table 6 SPADI	
How severe is your pain?	
1. At its worst	*(No pain)* 0 1 2 3 4 5 6 7 8 9 10 *(worst pain imaginable)*
2. When lying on involved side	*(No pain)* 0 1 2 3 4 5 6 7 8 9 10 *(worst pain imaginable)*
3. Reaching for something on a high shelf	*(No pain)* 0 1 2 3 4 5 6 7 8 9 10 *(worst pain imaginable)*
4. Touching the back of your neck	*(No pain)* 0 1 2 3 4 5 6 7 8 9 10 *(worst pain imaginable)*
5. Pushing with the involved arm	*(No pain)* 0 1 2 3 4 5 6 7 8 9 10 *(worst pain imaginable)*
How much difficulty do you have?	
1. Washing your hair	*(No difficulty)* 0 1 2 3 4 5 6 7 8 9 10 *(so difficult help is required)*
2. Washing your back	*(No difficulty)* 0 1 2 3 4 5 6 7 8 9 10 *(so difficult help is required)*
3. Putting on an undershirt or pullover sweater	*(No difficulty)* 0 1 2 3 4 5 6 7 8 9 10 *(so difficult help is required)*
4. Putting on a shirt that buttons down the front	*(No difficulty)* 0 1 2 3 4 5 6 7 8 9 10 *(so difficult help is required)*
5. Putting on your pants	*(No difficulty)* 0 1 2 3 4 5 6 7 8 9 10 *(so difficult help is required)*
6. Placing an object on a high shelf	*(No difficulty)* 0 1 2 3 4 5 6 7 8 9 10 *(so difficult help is required)*
7. Carrying a heavy object of 10 pounds	*(No difficulty)* 0 1 2 3 4 5 6 7 8 9 10 *(so difficult help is required)*
8. Removing something from your back pocket	*(No difficulty)* 0 1 2 3 4 5 6 7 8 9 10 *(so difficult help is required)*

Scoring

Pain score:
_____/50 × 100 = ____%
Sum of numbers circled in pain section
Disability score:
_____/80 × 100 = ____%
Sum of numbers circled in disability section

Total score:
_____/130 × 100 = ____%
Sum of numbers circled in both sections

From Roach KE, Budiman-Mak E, Songsiridej N, et al. Development of a shoulder pain and disability index. Arthritis Care Res 1991;4(4):143–9; with permission.

patients' work tasks, their injury, and their response to rehabilitation. Typically, factors such as lifting, pulling, and repetitive overhead work require modifications in position, force, repetitions, and/or duration. Those workers returning to jobs with heavy lifting or prolonged overhead work may need additional weeks of rehabilitation to regain full strength.

FUNCTIONAL DISABILITY SCALES FOR SHOULDER CONDITIONS

The SST and the SPADI are publically available and free of charge. They are reproduced in **Tables 5** and **6**.

The DASH and *Quick*DASH can be obtained by individual clinicians from the Institute for Work and Health (http://www.dash.iwh.on.ca/).

The ASES also has a measurement tool that is proprietary.

ACKNOWLEDGMENTS

Labor and Industries' Industrial Insurance Medical Advisory Committee (IIMAC) and its subcommittee on shoulder conditions developed this guideline in 2013. Acknowledgment and gratitude go to all subcommittee members, clinical experts, and consultants who contributed to this important guideline:

IIMAC committee members: Andrew Friedman MD; Chris Howe MD, Chair; Gerald Yorioka MD; Karen Nilson MD; Kirk Harmon MD.

Subcommittee clinical experts: Michael Codsi MD; Eric Fletcher PT; Laura Rachel Kaufman MD.

Consultation provided by Ken O'Bara MD, Qualis Health; Shari Fowler-Koorn RN, Qualis Health; Mike Dowling DC.

Department staff who helped develop and prepare this guideline include Gary M. Franklin MD MPH, Medical Director; Lee Glass MD, Associate Medical Director; Hal Stockbridge MD MPH, Associate Medical Director; Robert Mootz DC, Associate Medical Director; Teresa Cooper MN, MPH, Occupational Nurse Consultant; Bintu Marong MS, Epidemiologist.

REFERENCES

1. Walker-Bone K, Cooper C. Hard work never hurt anyone–or did it? A review of occupational associations with soft tissue musculoskeletal disorders of the neck and upper limb. Ann Rheum Dis 2005;64(8):1112–7.
2. Tashjian RZ. Epidemiology, natural history, and indications for treatment of rotator cuff tears. Clin Sports Med 2012;31(4):589–604.
3. Ottenheijm RP, Jansen MJ, Staal JB, et al. Accuracy of diagnostic ultrasound in patients with suspected subacromial disorders: a systematic review and meta-analysis. Arch Phys Med Rehabil 2010;91(10):1616–25.
4. Dinnes J, Loveman E, McIntyre L, et al. The effectiveness of diagnostic tests for the assessment of shoulder pain due to soft tissue disorders: a systematic review. Health Technol Assess 2003;7:iii, 1-166.
5. Vlychou M, Dailiana Z, Fotiadou A, et al. Symptomatic partial rotator cuff tears: diagnostic performance of ultrasound and magnetic resonance imaging with surgical correlation. Acta Radiol 2009;50(1):101–5.
6. de Jesus JO, Parker L, Frangos AJ, et al. Accuracy of MRI, MR arthrography, and ultrasound in the diagnosis of rotator cuff tears: a meta-analysis. AJR Am J Roentgenol 2009;192(6):1701–7.

7. Teefey SA, Rubin DA, Middleton WD, et al. Detection and quantification of rotator cuff tears. Comparison of ultrasonographic, magnetic resonance imaging, and arthroscopic findings in seventy-one consecutive cases. J Bone Joint Surg Am 2004;86-A(4):708–16.

8. Fallahi F, Green N, Gadde S, et al. Indirect magnetic resonance arthrography of the shoulder; a reliable diagnostic tool for investigation of suspected labral pathology. Skeletal Radiol 2013;42(9):1225–33.

9. Waldt S, Burkart A, Lange P, et al. Diagnostic performance of MR arthrography in the assessment of superior labral anteroposterior lesions of the shoulder. AJR Am J Roentgenol 2004;182(5):1271–8.

10. Buchbinder R, Green S, Youd JM, et al. Oral steroids for adhesive capsulitis. Cochrane Database Syst Rev 2006;(4):CD006189.

11. Brantingham JW, Cassa TK, Bonnefin D, et al. Manipulative therapy for shoulder pain and disorders: expansion of a systematic review. J Manipulative Physiol Ther 2011;34(5):314–46.

12. Littlewood C, Ashton J, Chance-Larsen K, et al. Exercise for rotator cuff tendinopathy: a systematic review. Physiotherapy 2012;98(2):101–9.

13. Marinko LN, Chacko JM, Dalton D, et al. The effectiveness of therapeutic exercise for painful shoulder conditions: a meta-analysis. J Shoulder Elbow Surg 2011; 20(8):1351–9.

14. Kuhn JE. Exercise in the treatment of rotator cuff impingement: a systematic review and a synthesized evidence-based rehabilitation protocol. J Shoulder Elbow Surg 2009;18(1):138–60.

15. Ryans I, Montgomery A, Galway R, et al. A randomized controlled trial of intra-articular triamcinolone and/or physiotherapy in shoulder capsulitis. Rheumatology (Oxford) 2005;44(4):529–35.

16. Calis M, Demir H, Ulker S, et al. Is intraarticular sodium hyaluronate injection an alternative treatment in patients with adhesive capsulitis? Rheumatol Int 2006; 26(6):536–40.

17. Tveita EK, Tariq R, Sesseng S, et al. Hydrodilatation, corticosteroids and adhesive capsulitis: a randomized controlled trial. BMC Musculoskelet Disord 2008; 9:53.

18. Rutten MJ, Maresch BJ, Jager GJ, et al. Injection of the subacromial-subdeltoid bursa: blind or ultrasound-guided? Acta Orthop 2007;78(2):254–7.

19. MacEachen E, Kosny A, Ferrier S, et al. The "toxic dose" of system problems: why some injured workers don't return to work as expected. J Occup Rehabil 2010; 20(3):349–66.

20. Pillastrini P, Mugnai R, Farneti C, et al. Evaluation of two preventive interventions for reducing musculoskeletal complaints in operators of video display terminals. Phys Ther 2007;87(5):536–44.

21. Rempel DM, Krause N, Goldberg R, et al. A randomised controlled trial evaluating the effects of two workstation interventions on upper body pain and incident musculoskeletal disorders among computer operators. Occup Environ Med 2006;63(5):300–6.

22. Godfrey J, Hamman R, Lowenstein S, et al. Reliability, validity, and responsiveness of the simple shoulder test: psychometric properties by age and injury type. J Shoulder Elbow Surg 2007;16(3):260–7.

23. MacDermid JC, Solomon P, Prkachin K. The shoulder pain and disability index demonstrates factor, construct and longitudinal validity. BMC Musculoskelet Disord 2006;7:12.

24. Angst F, Goldhahn J, Pap G, et al. Cross-cultural adaptation, reliability and validity of the German Shoulder Pain and Disability Index (SPADI). Rheumatology (Oxford) 2007;46(1):87–92.

25. Gabel CP, Yelland M, Melloh M, et al. A modified QuickDASH-9 provides a valid outcome instrument for upper limb function. BMC Musculoskelet Disord 2009;10:161.

26. Roy JS, MacDermid JC, Woodhouse LJ. Measuring shoulder function: a systematic review of four questionnaires. Arthritis Rheum 2009;61(5):623–32.

27. Beaton DE, Wright JG, Katz JN. Development of the QuickDASH: comparison of three item-reduction approaches. J Bone Joint Surg Am 2005;87(5): 1038–46.

28. Gummesson C, Ward MM, Atroshi I. The shortened disabilities of the arm, shoulder and hand questionnaire (QuickDASH): validity and reliability based on responses within the full-length DASH. BMC Musculoskelet Disord 2006;7:44.

29. Yamamoto A, Takagishi K, Osawa T, et al. Prevalence and risk factors of a rotator cuff tear in the general population. J Shoulder Elbow Surg 2010;19(1):116–20.

30. Baumgarten KM, Gerlach D, Galatz LM, et al. Cigarette smoking increases the risk for rotator cuff tears. Clin Orthop Relat Res 2010;468(6):1534–41.

31. Park HB, Yokota A, Gill HS, et al. Diagnostic accuracy of clinical tests for the different degrees of subacromial impingement syndrome. J Bone Joint Surg Am 2005;87:1446–55.

32. Gazzola S, Bleakney RR. Current imaging of the rotator cuff. Sports Med Arthrosc 2011;19(3):300–9.

33. Safran O, Schroeder J, Bloom R, et al. Natural history of nonoperatively treated symptomatic rotator cuff tears in patients 60 years old or younger. Am J Sports Med 2011;39(4):710–4.

34. Mall NA, Kim HM, Keener JD, et al. Symptomatic progression of asymptomatic rotator cuff tears: a prospective study of clinical and sonographic variables. J Bone Joint Surg Am 2010;92(16):2623–33.

35. Yamaguchi K, Sher JS, Andersen WK, et al. Glenohumeral motion in patients with rotator cuff tears: a comparison of asymptomatic and symptomatic shoulders. J Shoulder Elbow Surg 2000;9(1):6–11.

36. Keener JD, Wei AS, Kim HM, et al. Proximal humeral migration in shoulders with symptomatic and asymptomatic rotator cuff tears. J Bone Joint Surg Am 2009; 91(6):1405–13.

37. Ejnisman B, Andreoli CV, Soares BG, et al. Interventions for tears of the rotator cuff in adults. Cochrane Database Syst Rev 2004;(1):CD002758.

38. Milano G, Grasso A, Salvatore M, et al. Arthroscopic rotator cuff repair with and without subacromial decompression: a prospective randomized study. Arthroscopy 2007;23(1):81–8.

39. Gartsman GM, O'Connor DP. Arthroscopic rotator cuff repair with and without arthroscopic subacromial decompression: a prospective, randomized study of one-year outcomes. J Shoulder Elbow Surg 2004;13(4):424–6.

40. Shin SJ, Oh JH, Chung SW, et al. The efficacy of acromioplasty in the arthroscopic repair of small- to medium-sized rotator cuff tears without acromial spur: prospective comparative study. Arthroscopy 2012;28(5):628–35.

41. MacDonald P, McRae S, Leiter J, et al. Arthroscopic rotator cuff repair with and without acromioplasty in the treatment of full-thickness rotator cuff tears: a multicenter, randomized controlled trial. J Bone Joint Surg Am 2011; 93(21):1953–60.

42. Phipatanakul WP, Petersen SA. Porcine small intestine submucosa xenograft augmentation in repair of massive rotator cuff tears. Am J Orthop (Belle Mead NJ) 2009;38(11):572–5.
43. Carbone S, Gumina S, Arceri V, et al. The impact of preoperative smoking habit on rotator cuff tear: cigarette smoking influences rotator cuff tear sizes. J Shoulder Elbow Surg 2012;21(1):56–60.
44. Galatz LM, Silva MJ, Rothermich SY, et al. Nicotine delays tendon-to-bone healing in a rat shoulder model. J Bone Joint Surg Am 2006;88(9):2027–34.
45. Mallon WJ, Misamore G, Snead DS, et al. The impact of preoperative smoking habits on the results of rotator cuff repair. J Shoulder Elbow Surg 2004;13(2):129–32.
46. Djurasovic M, Marra G, Arroyo JS, et al. Revision rotator cuff repair: factors influencing results. J Bone Joint Surg Am 2001;83-A(12):1849–55.
47. van Rijn RM, Huisstede BM, Koes BW, et al. Associations between work-related factors and specific disorders of the shoulder–a systematic review of the literature. Scand J Work Environ Health 2010;36(3):189–201.
48. Haahr JP, Andersen JH. Exercises may be as efficient as subacromial decompression in patients with subacromial stage II impingement: 4-8-years' follow-up in a prospective, randomized study. Scand J Rheumatol 2006;35(3):224–8.
49. Haahr JP, Ostergaard S, Dalsgaard J, et al. Exercises versus arthroscopic decompression in patients with subacromial impingement: a randomised, controlled study in 90 cases with a one year follow up. Ann Rheum Dis 2005; 64(5):760–4.
50. Gosens T, Hofstee DJ. Calcifying tendinitis of the shoulder: advances in imaging and management. Curr Rheumatol Rep 2009;11(2):129–34.
51. Oliva F, Via AG, Maffulli N. Physiopathology of intratendinous calcific deposition. BMC Med 2012;10:95.
52. Uhthoff H. Anatomopathology of calcifying tendinitis of the cuff. In: Gazielly DF, Gleyze PTT, editors. The cuff. Paris: Elsevier; 1997.
53. Lam F, Bhatia D, Van Rooyen K, et al. Modern management of calcifying tendinitis of the shoulder. Curr Orthop 2006;20(6):446–52.
54. Rockwood CA, Williams GR, Youg DC. Disorders of the acromioclavicular joint. In: Rockwood CA, Masten FA II, editors. The shoulder. Philadelphia: Saunders; 1998. p. 483–553.
55. Brockmeier SF, Voos JE, Williams RJ 3rd, et al. Outcomes after arthroscopic repair of type-II SLAP lesions. J Bone Joint Surg Am 2009;91(7):1595–603.
56. Mileski RA, Snyder SJ. Superior labral lesions in the shoulder: pathoanatomy and surgical management. J Am Acad Orthop Surg 1998;6(2):121–31.
57. Bedi A, Allen AA. Superior labral lesions anterior to posterior-evaluation and arthroscopic management. Clin Sports Med 2008;27(4):607–30.
58. Magee T, Williams D, Mani N. Shoulder MR arthrography: which patient group benefits most? AJR Am J Roentgenol 2004;183(4):969–74.
59. Jee WH, McCauley TR, Katz LD, et al. Superior labral anterior posterior (SLAP) lesions of the glenoid labrum: reliability and accuracy of MR arthrography for diagnosis. Radiology 2001;218(1):127–32.
60. Phillips JC, Cook C, Beaty S, et al. Validity of noncontrast magnetic resonance imaging in diagnosing superior labrum anterior-posterior tears. J Shoulder Elbow Surg 2013;22(1):3–8.
61. Amin MF, Youssef AO. The diagnostic value of magnetic resonance arthrography of the shoulder in detection and grading of SLAP lesions: comparison with arthroscopic findings. Eur J Radiol 2012;81(9):2343–7.

62. Provencher MT, McCormick F, Dewing C, et al. A prospective analysis of 179 type 2 superior labrum anterior and posterior repairs: outcomes and factors associated with success and failure. Am J Sports Med 2013;41:880–6.

63. Koh KH, Ahn JH, Kim SM, et al. Treatment of biceps tendon lesions in the setting of rotator cuff tears: prospective cohort study of tenotomy versus tenodesis. Am J Sports Med 2010;38(8):1584–90.

64. Franceschi F, Longo UG, Ruzzini L, et al. No advantages in repairing a type II superior labrum anterior and posterior (SLAP) lesion when associated with rotator cuff repair in patients over age 50: a randomized controlled trial. Am J Sports Med 2008;36(2):247–53.

65. Kaisidis A, Pantos P, Heger H, et al. Arthroscopic fixation of isolated type II SLAP lesions using a two-portal technique. Acta Orthop Belg 2011;77(2): 160–6.

66. Alpert JM, Wuerz TH, O'Donnell TF, et al. The effect of age on the outcomes of arthroscopic repair of type II superior labral anterior and posterior lesions. Am J Sports Med 2010;38(11):2299–303.

67. Chahal J, Marks PH, Macdonald PB, et al. Anatomic Bankart repair compared with nonoperative treatment and/or arthroscopic lavage for first-time traumatic shoulder dislocation. Arthroscopy 2012;28(4):565–75.

68. Robinson CM, Jenkins PJ, White TO, et al. Primary arthroscopic stabilization for a first-time anterior dislocation of the shoulder. A randomized, double-blind trial. J Bone Joint Surg Am 2008;90(4):708–21.

69. Harris JD, Gupta AK, Mall NA, et al. Long-term outcomes after Bankart shoulder stabilization. Arthroscopy 2013;29(5):920–33.

70. Fabbriciani C, Milano G, Demontis A, et al. Arthroscopic versus open treatment of Bankart lesion of the shoulder: a prospective randomized study. Arthroscopy 2004;20(5):456–62.

71. D'Alessandro DF, Bradley JP, Fleischli JE, et al. Prospective evaluation of thermal capsulorrhaphy for shoulder instability: indications and results, two- to five-year follow-up. Am J Sports Med 2004;32(1):21–33.

72. Slenker NR, Lawson K, Ciccotti MG, et al. Biceps tenotomy versus tenodesis: clinical outcomes. Arthroscopy 2012;28(4):576–82.

73. Kelly AM, Drakos MC, Fealy S, et al. Arthroscopic release of the long head of the biceps tendon: functional outcome and clinical results. Am J Sports Med 2005; 33(2):208–13.

APPENDIX: SPECIFIC SHOULDER TEST

Rotator cuff impingement

- The *Neer* test assesses for possible rotator cuff impingement. Stabilize the scapula (place your hand firmly on the acromion or hold the inferior angle of the scapula with your hand); with the thumb pointing down, passively flex the arm. Pain is a positive test.

- The *Hawkins* test assesses for possible rotator cuff impingement. Stabilize the scapula; passively abduct the shoulder to 90°; flex the shoulder to 30°; flex the elbow to 90°; internally rotate the shoulder. Pain is a positive test.

Rotator cuff tears

- Abduction test: Perform active abduction to 90° while providing resistance proximal to the elbow (primary abductor: supraspinatus).

- External rotation test: Examiner places one hand on the medial elbow and the other on the lateral aspect of the distal forearm. Instruct the patient to externally rotate the shoulder while you provide resistance. It is important to stabilize the patient's elbow against their side to prevent them from substituting abduction for external rotation. Compare the strength of the involved shoulder with that of the uninvolved shoulder. This test may also elicit pain indicating inflammation and weakness in the external rotators (primary external rotator: infraspinatus).

- *Lateral Jobe test*: Patients hold their arm at 90° abduction in the coronal plane with elbows flexed at 90° and hands pointing inferiorly with the thumbs directed medially. A positive test consists of pain or weakness on resisting downward pressure on the arms or an inability to perform the tests.

AC joint test

- *Crossed arm adduction*: Flex the shoulder to 90° and adduct the arm across the body (reaching for opposite shoulder). Pain at the AC joint is a positive test.

Labral tears, tendon disorders, dislocations

- The *O'Brien test:* Point the thumb down. Flex the shoulder to 90° and adduct the arm across midline. Provide resistance against further shoulder flexion and evaluate for pain. Repeat with thumb pointing up and again evaluate for pain. If pain was present with the thumb down but relieved with the thumb up, it is considered a positive test, suspicious for a labral tear.

- The *Yergason* test: Flex the elbow to 90°, shake hands with patient and provide resistance against supination. Pain indicates possible bicipital tendinopathy or a labral tear.

- The *Speed* test: Flex the shoulder to 90° with the arm supinated. Provide downward resistance against shoulder flexion. Pain indicates possible bicipital tendinopathy or a labral tear.

- *Biceps load* test: Supinate the arm; abduct the shoulder to 90°; flex the elbow to 90°; externally rotate the arm until patients become apprehensive and provide resistance against elbow flexion. Pain indicates possible bicipital tendinopathy or a labral tear.

- *Apprehension* test: It evaluates for anterior glenohumeral stability. With patients supine, abduct the shoulder to 90° and externally rotate the arm to place stress on the glenohumeral joint. If patients feel apprehension that the arm may dislocate anteriorly, the test is positive. The apprehension test is usually followed by the relocation test: with the hand, place a posteriorly directed force on the glenohumeral joint. Relief of apprehension for dislocation is a positive test.

http://www.shoulderdoc.co.uk/article.asp?section=497

http://at.uwa.edu/special%20tests/specialtests/UpperBody/shoulder%20Main%20Page.htm

http://sitemaker.umich.edu/fm_musculoskeletal_shoulder/shoulder_exam_manuevers

Diagnosis and Treatment of Cervical Radiculopathy and Myelopathy

Jean-Christophe A. Leveque, MD[a], Bintu Marong-Ceesay, MS[b], Teresa Cooper, MN, MPH[c], Chris R. Howe, MD[d],*

KEYWORDS

- Cervical • Radiculopathy • Myelopathy • Anterior cervical discectomy and fusion
- Foraminotomy

KEY POINTS

- The surgical treatment of degenerative discs is generally discouraged.
- Symptomatic cervical radiculopathies can improve with nonoperative management.
- The decision to pursue surgery, or surgical consultation, is appropriate when myelopathic symptoms are present.

INTRODUCTION

The following guideline is intended as a community standard for health care providers who treat injured workers or others with symptomatic cervical pathology. The guideline aims to help ensure that the diagnosis and treatment of cervical neck conditions are of the highest quality. The emphasis is on accurate diagnosis and curative or rehabilitative treatment.

The recommendations are based on the best available clinical and scientific evidence from a systematic review of the literature, and on a consensus of expert opinion when scientific evidence was insufficient. The following table summarizes the recommendations:

CERVICAL SURGERY REVIEW CRITERIA

Disclosures: None.
[a] Group Health, Seattle, Washington, USA; [b] Department of Health, Olympia, Washington, USA; [c] Department of Labor and Industries, Olympia, Washington, USA; [d] Proliance Orthopedic Associates, Renton, Washington, USA
* Corresponding author. Proliance Orthopedic Associates, 4011 Talbot Road South, Suite #300, Renton, WA 98055, USA.
E-mail address: c.howe@proliancesurgeons.com

Phys Med Rehabil Clin N Am 26 (2015) 491–511
http://dx.doi.org/10.1016/j.pmr.2015.04.008
1047-9651/15/$ – see front matter © 2015 Elsevier Inc. All rights reserved.

pmr.theclinics.com

A Request May Be Appropriate for	And the Diagnosis Is Supported by These Clinical Findings			And This Has Been Done (if Recommended)
Surgical Procedure & Diagnosis	Subjective	Objective	Imaging	Conservative Care
Surgery (in general) for: neck pain without subjective, objective, and imaging evidence of radiculopathy or myelopathy	Surgery is not recommended (the surgical treatment of disc degeneration or facet arthropathy without an associated radiculopathy or myelopathy is not well established in the literature and is generally contraindicated			
Surgery (in general) for: neck pain without subjective, objective, and imaging evidence of radiculopathy or myelopathy				
ACDF, TDA, laminotomy, foraminotomy for: radiculopathy single level	Sensory symptoms (radicular pain and/or paresthesias) in a dermatomal distribution that correlates with involved cervical level **AND**	Motor deficit **OR** Reflex changes **OR** Positive EMG Findings should correlate with involved cervical level **AND**	MRI **OR** Myelogram with computed tomography (CT) scan Abnormal imaging read by radiologist (moderate-to-severe foraminal stenosis) that correlates nerve root involvement with subjective and objective findings **AND** In the case of discordant reading between surgeon and radiologist, an independent radiologist opinion is needed	At least 6 weeks[a] of conservative care, such as: • Physical therapy emphasizing active modalities • Osteopathic manipulation • Chiropractic manipulation • Anti-inflammatory medication • Epidural injections **AND** [a]In the case of clear motor deficit after an acute injury, the 6 weeks of conservative care are not required
		OR		
	Sensory symptoms (radicular pain and/or paresthesias) in a dermatomal distribution that correlates with involved cervical level		A positive response to a selective nerve root block, as determined and documented by the interventionist, in the case of complaints of radicular pain without motor, sensory, reflex or EMG changes. Criteria for selective nerve root blocks (see page 9 for details): • Use low-volume(≤1.0 cc) local anesthetic, with fluoroscopy or CT scan • No sedation should be given with SNRB, except in extreme cases of anxiety • Document a baseline level of pain • Meaningful improvement in pain (80% improvement from pre-block baseline, or 5-point change on VAS) • Only one level of surgery will be approved if SNRB is the sole basis for objective diagnosis	

ACDF, TDA, laminotomy, foraminotomy, or corpectomy for: radiculopathy—2 levels	A 2-level surgery may be considered if the following criteria are met: All of the criteria previously described for single-level fusion (not including SNRB) are present at the primary level, AND • The adjacent level has radicular pain correlating with at least moderate foraminal stenosis or lateral recess herniation, OR • EMG changes, muscle weakness, or reflex changes that indicate involvement of the adjacent level If the first level has no findings except the response to SNRB, a second level is generally not recommended Total disc arthroplasty is contraindicated in the presence of moderate-to-severe facet arthropathy or measurable instability (>3.5mm) and/or >11° of rotational difference to either adjacent level
ACDF, laminotomy, foraminotomy, or corpectomy for: radiculopathy-3 or more	All the objective criteria previously described for single-level radiculopathy, which does not include SNRBs, must be met for each level for which surgery is being requested
ACDF, laminotomy, foraminotomy, or corpectomy for: adjacent segment pathology	There is insufficient evidence in the medical literature to support a causal link between symptomatic adjacent segment pathology and cervical fusion; therefore, treatment for ASP should generally not be accepted in workers' compensation claims, unless there is compelling radiographic evidence that previous surgery has directly compromised (eg, hardware displacement) the adjacent segment

ACDF, TDA, laminectomy ± fusion, or corpectomy for: myelopathy, single-level	History of: Hand clumsiness or incoordination, gait disturbance, bowel or bladder dysfunction,	A combination of abnormal lower and upper motor neuron findings in upper extremities OR Upper motor neuron signs in the lower extremities Examples: • Loss of fine motor control • Weakness • Hand clumsiness • Gait disturbance • Bowel or bladder dysfunction • Increased tone in arms and/or legs • Hyperactive reflexes including Hoffman sign and/or clonus	Myelogram with CT scan OR MRI Abnormal imaging that correlates with subjective and objective findings: AND Cord signal change OR Compression with loss of circumferential CSF signal OR Stenosis (≤8mm AP diameter) In the case of discordant reading between surgeon and radiologist, an independent radiology opinion is recommended	Not required if there is evidence of myelopathy

AND ... AND

ACDF, laminectomy ±fusion, laminoplasty, corpectomy for: myelopathy, multilevel	If the criteria previously described, including imaging findings, are met for single-level myelopathy, the levels of surgical intervention are generally deferred to the surgeon given the complexity of surgical decision making				
Repeat surgery for: pseudarthrosis	Axial neck pain	AND	No definitive physical examination findings	CT finding of nonunion (after 1 year or more) OR Hardware failure OR Flexion/extension radiographs showing >2 mm of interspinous motion. AND CT SPECT if previously described findings not definitive	Repeat surgery for pseudarthrosis is generally not considered until 1 year after original surgery
Repeat Surgeries at same level not due to pseudarthrosis	All the criteria described previously for single-level radiculopathy must be met Consideration for repeat surgeries should proceed with considerable caution; there should be documented and substantial improvement in pain and function on a validated instrument after the first surgery before a second surgery will be approved or a clear documented reason for lack of improvement after the initial procedure				
Hybrid Surgeries (defined as a ACDF next to a TDA)	The department considers hybrid procedures to be investigational. There is insufficient evidence in medical literature to permit conclusions on its safety and efficacy				

Abbreviations: ACDF, anterior cervical discectomy and fusion; AP, anteroposterior; ASP, adjacent segment pathology; CSF, cerebrospinal fluid; EMG, electromyography; SPECT, single-photon emission computed tomography; SNRB, selective nerve root block; TDA, total disc arthoplasty; VAS, visual analogue scale.

[a] For nicotine users: Abstinence from nicotine is recommended for all fusions and repeat fusions done for radiculopathy. This does not apply to progressive myelopathy or motor radiculopathy.

BACKGROUND AND PREVALENCE

Neck-related pain is common in both the workers' compensation and general populations. Many cases of axial neck pain are temporary and will resolve with time and nonoperative treatment.[1] It can be difficult to distinguish between an acute or chronic condition related to work and the chronic pain and degeneration associated with aging.

Cervical degenerative disc disease (DDD) is a common cause of pain and disability, affecting approximately two-thirds of the US adult population.[1] Most symptomatic cases present between the ages of 40 and 60,[2] although many individuals never develop symptoms. MRI studies have documented the presence of DDD in 60% of asymptomatic individuals aged greater than 40 years and 80% of patients over the age of 80 years (**Figs. 1** and **2**).[3,4] Previous neck injuries, cervical strains, and arthritis increase the risk of developing DDD, which may result in the development of abnormal bony spurs (spondylosis). Less commonly, cervical DDD progression and its sequelae may directly compress parts of the spinal cord (myelopathy), affecting gait and balance. It may also result in foraminal narrowing, compressing the exiting nerve root (radiculopathy), resulting in a dermatomal distribution of numbness, pain or paresthesias, or a myotomal distribution of weakness (**Figs. 3** and **4**).

Treatment options for DDD include conservative and surgical measures. In the general population, the rate of surgery for degenerative disc disease of the cervical spine increased 90% between 1990 and 2000.[5] In elderly patients in the United States, rates of cervical fusions rose 206% between 1992 and 2005.[6] Annual costs for anterior cervical fusions increased 3 fold ($1.62 billion to $5.63 billion) between 2000 and 2009.[7]

ESTABLISHING WORK-RELATEDNESS

The etiology of radiculopathies and myelopathies can be multifactorial or unknown. A cervical condition presenting with a history of radiating arm pain, scapular pain,

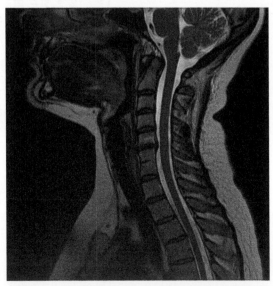

Fig. 1. Sagittal magnetic resonance image demonstrating mild degenerative cervical changes at C5/6 in a patient with moderate neck pain but no radicular or myelopathic syptoms.

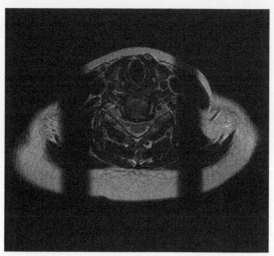

Fig. 2. Axial magnetic resonance image in the same patient showing disc bulging but no central or foraminal stenosis.

diminished muscle stretch reflexes, loss of sensation, or motor weakness may be classified as an occupational injury or occupational disease depending upon the circumstances giving rise to the condition. If there was a single inciting event that occurred within the work environment resulting in objective medical findings, the condition is likely the result of an occupational injury. If there was no single inciting event, the condition may have risen as the result of an occupational disease. The pain and other manifestations of both industrial injuries and occupational diseases generally become

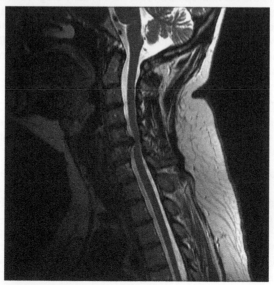

Fig. 3. Sagittal magnetic resonance image demonstrating a large focal disc herniation at the C5/6 level causing radicular pain and weakness.

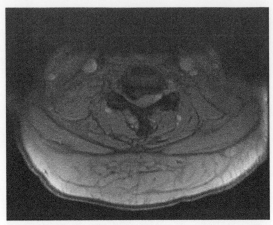

Fig. 4. Axial magnetic resonance image in the same patient demonstrating a large right C5/6 disc herniation with severe foraminal narrowing.

evident within 3 months of the inciting event. For this reason, a condition reported for the first time more than 3 months after a patient was first seen by a provider may not be industrially related. Attribution of such a condition to an industrial event should be based upon careful analysis and thoroughly documented.

Cervical Conditions as Industrial Injuries

Mechanisms of injury to the cervical spine may include distortion of the neck caused by sudden movement of the head, being struck by an object, or a fall from a height.[8–10] Examples of these injuries include motor vehicle crashes, high impact accidents, explosions, and gunshots.[11–13]

An acute injury to the cervical spine should be clinically diagnosable as work-related within 3 months of the injury. For an injury claim to the neck to be accepted beyond 3 months, the attending provider should be able to present substantial evidence linking symptoms directly to the initial industrial injury. Claims with insufficient documentation linking clinical symptoms to the initial industrial injury beyond 1 year should generally not be accepted.

Cervical Conditions as Occupational Diseases

Cervical spine conditions may also develop as a natural consequence of aging, resulting in the deterioration of the cervical disc. To establish a diagnosis of an occupational disease all of the following are required:

1. Exposure—workplace activities that contribute to or cause cervical spine conditions
2. Outcome—a diagnosis of a cervical spine condition that meets the diagnostic criteria in this guideline
3. Relationship—for a cervical condition to be allowed as an occupational disease, the provider must document that, based on generally accepted scientific evidence, the work exposures created a risk of contracting or worsening the condition relative to the risks in everyday life, on a more-probable-than-not basis (*Dennis v. Dept. of Labor and Industries*, 1987).[14] In epidemiologic studies, this will usually translate to an odds ratio (OR) of at least 2.

MAKING THE DIAGNOSIS
History and Clinical Examination

The classic presentation of cervical radiculopathy includes radiating arm pain, scapular pain, diminished muscle stretch reflexes, loss of sensation, and motor weakness, with or without neck pain. Cervical myelopathy is characterized by loss of motor control, hand clumsiness, gait disturbances, spasticity, and bowel or bladder dysfunction.

Diagnostic Testing—Imaging/Myelogram/Electromyographys

Requirements for diagnostic testing and imaging are specified in the criteria table. The basis for the selection of a diagnostic imaging procedure should be based on the information obtained from a thorough clinical examination.

Selective Nerve Root Blocks

Selective nerve root blocks (SNRBs) are only considered criteria for surgery when a worker presents with radicular pain, imaging findings, and a history of 6 weeks of conservative care (as in the criteria table), but does not have the objective signs of motor, reflex or EMG changes. SNRBs should be used only under particular circumstances:

- The worker has clear sensory symptoms indicative of radiculopathy or nerve root irritation.
- The worker's symptoms and examination findings are consistent with injury or irritation of the nerve root that is to be blocked.
- Injury or irritation of the nerve root to be blocked has not been shown to exist by electrodiagnostic, imaging, or other studies.

It is recommended that the provider giving the injection has the principal responsibility to document the outcome of the selective nerve root block. The provider should

- Perform a preinjection examination and document the pain intensity using a validated scale
- Explain to the worker the use and importance of the postinjection pain diary
- Use low-volume local anesthetic (≤1.0 cc) without steroid for the selective nerve root block; conscious sedation should not be used in the administration of SNRBs, except in cases of extreme anxiety. If sedation is used, the reason(s) must be documented in the medical record, and the record must be furnished to the department or self-insurer
- Administer the selective nerve root block using fluoroscopic or computed tomography (CT) guidance. An archival image of the injection procedure must be produced, and a copy must be provided to the department or self-insurer (**Fig. 5**).
- Onset (within 1 hour) of pain relief should be consistent with the anesthetic used; duration generally lasting 2 to 4 hours.
- Keep the worker in the office for 15 to 30 minutes after the injection if possible, and assist with starting the pain diary.
  ○ Immediately preceding the block, the worker should record the level of pain using a validated scale. Every 15 minutes thereafter, for at least 6 hours following injection, the worker should indicate his or her level of pain. For the remaining waking hours during the 24 hours following the administration of the block, hourly documentation of pain levels is desirable.
  ○ An example of a pain diary is included in this guideline. Pain must be measured and documented using validated tools such as a visual analog scale or a 10-point scale. See labor and industries (L&I's) opioid prescribing guideline

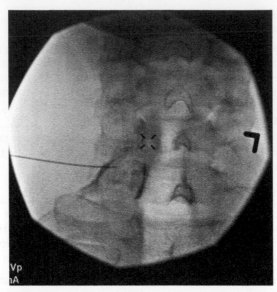

Fig. 5. Fluoroscopic image during a selective nerve root block demonstrating contrast dye outlining the region of injection along the C7 nerve.

(www.opioids.LNI.WA.GOV) for a 2-item graded chronic pain scale, which is a valid measure of pain and pain interference with function.
- Document the effect of the block.
  - A positive block is indicated by
    - An overall 80% improvement in pain or pain reduction by at least 5 points on a 10-point scale or visual analog scale
    - Pain relief that lasts an amount of time consistent with the duration of the anesthetic used
  - A negative block may be indicated by
    - No pain relief or less than 5 points on a 10-point scale or visual analog scale
    - Pain relief that is inconsistent in duration with the usual mechanism of action of the local anesthetic given
- Ensure that the surgeon and the department or self-insurer receive the previously described information.

If the block is negative, surgery is generally not recommended. Only 1 level of surgery should be considered if the sole basis of the objective diagnosis is the SNRB.

TREATMENT
Conservative Treatment

Conservative management of cervical radicular symptoms may include active physical therapy, osteopathic manipulation, chiropractic manipulation, traction, nonsteroidal anti-inflammatory drugs (NSAIDs) and steroid injections.

- There is some evidence that an active treatment approach results in better outcomes.[15,16] Physical therapy accompanied by home exercise for 6 weeks has been shown in a randomized trial to substantially reduce neck and arm pain for patients with cervical radiculopathy.[17]

- Steroid injections may provide short-term pain relief for patients with radiculopathy,[18,19] although they are not without risks. The injection typically includes both steroid and a long-acting anesthetic. See Washington States L&I's guideline on spinal injections at http://www.lni.wa.gov/ClaimsIns/Providers/TreatingPatients/TreatGuide/spinal.asp.

> There is a warning about epidural steroid injections. On April 23, 2014, the US Food and Drug Administration (FDA) put out a warning that the injection of corticosteroids into the epidural space of the spine may result in rare but serious adverse events, including loss of vision, stroke, paralysis and death (FDA Drug Safety Communications 4-23-2014).[20]

Surgical Treatment

The ideal surgical approach for radiculopathy related to herniated disc remains a matter of debate. Various studies have compared the different surgery types and found no significant difference among them. Cervical surgeries can be divided into 2 major approaches: anterior (with or without fusion) and posterior.

Anterior cervical decompression alone

Discectomy is a surgical procedure to remove part of a herniated disc to alleviate pressure on the surrounding nerve roots. Discectomy is generally a safe procedure with associated risk such as dysphagia, pseudoarthrosis, and nerve damage. Studies, albeit dated, comparing discectomy with discectomy plus fusion have found no statistically significant difference between simple discectomy and discectomy followed by fusion in the treatment of cervical radiculopathy.[21–23]

Posterior surgeries

Posterior cervical laminotomy/foraminotomy is a highly effective therapeutic procedure for both myelopathy and radiculopathy, as it maintains cervical range of motion, and minimizes adjacent segment degeneration.[24–26] Kyphosis, incomplete neurologic decompression, and continued persistent neck pain have been concerns with posterior foraminotomies, but studies have shown it to be comparable to anterior cervical discectomy with fusion (ACDF) in clinical outcomes.[27–29]

Anterior cervical discectomy with fusion

Anterior cervical fusion surgery has become a standard treatment for cervical disc disease, and it is a proven intervention for patients with myelopathy and radiculopathy as it affords the surgeon the ability to provide direct (from the discectomy) and indirect (through restoration of disc height) decompression and stabilization.[30–32] Various implant and graft devices have been developed for use with ACDF.[21,22]

Total disc arthroplasty

Total disc arthroplasty (TDA) has been proposed as a viable alternative to ACDF. The theoretic basis for cervical arthroplasty is that it maintains motion and may decrease the likelihood of adjacent segment disease and therefore reduce the rate of reoperations.[33,34] Various studies have shown similar outcomes for ACDF and TDA.[35–37]

TDA is not indicated for cervical disease at more than 2 levels. Various devices have FDA approval for single-level TDA, and the FDA has also approved a single devise maker for 2-level adjacent disc arthroplasty in 2013. These devices are indicated for skeletally mature patients for reconstruction of disc following discectomy at a single level or adjacent (in the case of the Mobi-C) levels for radiculopathy or myelopathy.

Patients should have failed 6 weeks of conservative treatment or demonstrate progressive signs and symptoms.

Multilevel surgeries
For radiculopathy, a multilevel (2 levels or more) surgery may be considered if all of the criteria for a single-level surgery, not including SNRBs, are present at each level being considered for surgery. Multilevel fusion for myelopathy is more common and may be done if indications are met (**Figs. 6** and **7**).

A condition requiring at least 2 levels of surgery is unlikely to be a work-related injury or disease. All requests for 3 or more levels under a worker's compensation program should be pursued with caution.

Hybrid surgeries
Hybrid surgeries combine artificial disc replacements and anterior cervical discectomy with fusion at select vertebral bodies (adjacent or nonadjacent) in a single procedure. There is insufficient evidence in the medical literature to permit conclusions on its safety and efficacy. In general, hybrid procedures are considered experimental and investigational. New evidence will be examined as it becomes available.

Repeat surgeries
Request for repeat surgeries should be pursued with caution and on an individual basis. There should be documented and substantial improvement in pain and function on a validated instrument after the first surgery before a second surgery will be approved or clear documentation of the reason for failure of the initial procedure.

Intraoperative monitoring
Somatosensory evoked potentials (SSEP) and motor evoked potentials (MEP) are sometimes used in neurologic and spinal surgeries. The use of intraoperative

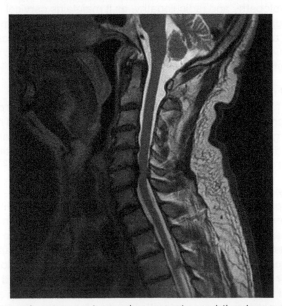

Fig. 6. Sagittal magnetic resonance image demonstrating multilevel central canal narrowing from C4/5 down through C6.

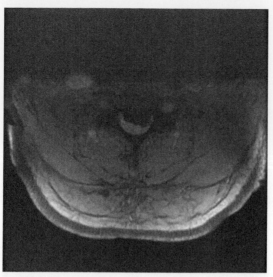

Fig. 7. Axial magnetic resonance image in the same patient demonstrating severe central canal narrowing at the C6 level.

neurophysiologic spinal cord monitoring is increasing despite a lack of consensus regarding accuracy, appropriate indications, and overall clinical benefits.[38–43]

The use of intraoperative monitoring for routine decompressive procedures (eg, discectomy or laminectomy) with or without fusion is generally discouraged. Intraoperative monitoring may be recommended for treatment of spinal deformities, traumatic dislocations, myelopathy, or posterior cervical instrumentation.[44]

Pseudarthrosis (non union)

Pseudarthrosis exists when there is a complete absence of bridging bone and either hardware failure or measurable instability. Symptomatic pseudarthrosis can be diagnosed based on clinical presentation and diagnostic imaging (**Fig. 8**). For a repeat surgery to be considered, CT SPECT or CT imaging showing nonincorporation of bone or flexion and extension radiograph showing interspinous motion greater than or equal to 2 mm is required.

A contributor to pseudarthrosis is smoking, as nicotine is a vasoconstrictor and also seems to block the ability of osteoblasts to form new bone.[45–47] Other patient-specific metabolic conditions such as diabetes may also contribute to nonunion.[48]

Smoking Cessation

Nicotine use is a strong contraindication to spine surgeries. Patients undergoing cervical fusions and repeat fusions for radiculopathy are required to abstain from nicotine for 4 weeks before surgery. In cases of myelopathy, smoking cessation is strongly encouraged but not required, since the progression of disease may preclude the time required for the patient to cease all nicotine-containing compounds.

ADJACENT SEGMENT PATHOLOGY

Adjacent segment degeneration, adjacent segment disease, and adjacent segment pathology (ASP) are terms commonly used to describe a degenerative pathology of the spine. The phenomenon of ASP is not fully understood. It has been predicted

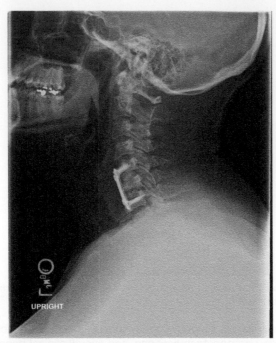

Fig. 8. Lateral radiograph of the cervical spine suggesting pseudoarthrosis at both operated levels, with bony nonunion and subsidence of the lower graft. Confirmation of pseudoarthrosis would require CT imaging.

that more than 25% of all patients would develop ASP during the first 10 years after ACDF.[49]

It remains unclear as to whether these conditions are related to altered biomechanics or represent the natural history of the cervical spine. It has been suggested that excessive motion of segments adjacent to a fixed fusion leads to an increased risk of disc degeneration. Fusion has been associated with ASP, but various studies have failed to show that it is an isolated factor.[50,51] Adjacent segment pathology has been seen after both anterior and posterior surgeries, as well as noninstrumented cases, suggesting that other factors may be involved in accelerating pathologic changes.[52,53]

ASP has been the driving force for the development of new alternative treatment methods such as TDA. These options were theoretically designed to be ideal substitutes for ACDF because of their motion-preserving benefits.[32,54] However, short-term studies comparing ACDF with TDA have failed to show any significant difference in the rate of adjacent segment disease following surgery.[37,55–62]

There is insufficient evidence in the medical literature to support a causal link between symptomatic adjacent segment pathology and cervical fusion. Therefore, treatment for ASP will generally not be accepted under a workers' compensation program unless there is compelling radiographic evidence that previous surgery has directly compromised (eg, hardware displacement) the adjacent segment (**Figs. 9–12**).

MEASURING FUNCTIONAL IMPROVEMENT

The goal of treatment is to improve pain and function. Providers should measure and document functional improvement throughout conservative and surgical treatment.

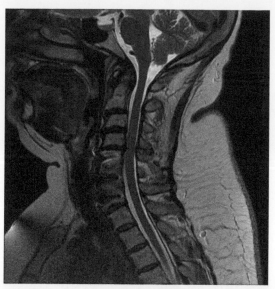

Fig. 9. Sagittal magnetic resonance image demonstrating C4/5 disc bulge in a patient with a previous C5/6 fusion. Further operative intervention at the C4/5 level would not be covered as adjacent segment failure.

Levels of pain must be documented when evaluating the results from SNRBs. Visual analog scales (VAS) or 0-point scales have been useful for this purpose. The 2-item graded chronic pain scale, as recommended in the L&I opioid prescribing guideline (http://lni.wa.gov/ClaimsIns/Files/OMD/MedTreat/FINALOpioidGuideline010713.pdf), is a simple way to document how much pain is interfering with function.

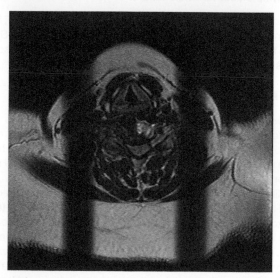

Fig. 10. Axial magnetic resonance image in the same patient demonstrating foraminal narrowing.

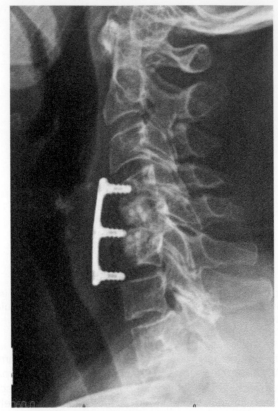

Fig. 11. Lateral radiograph image demonstrating a profound hardware failure and nonunion from a previous C fusion. Operative correction would generally be covered under the provision for symptomatic hardware failure.

The Neck Disability Index (NDI), Short Form Health Survey (SF)-36, SF-12, and VAS are tools recommended by the North American Spine Society (NASS) to assess pain and function and to measure outcome of treatment. Other validated scales and instruments may be used to document improvement or lack thereof.

POSTOPERATIVE PHASE AND RETURN TO WORK

It is important for the attending provider and the surgeon to focus on preoperative planning for postoperative recovery, reactivation, and return to work activities. During the immediate postoperative period, (6 weeks), the surgeon should help direct these activities. It is the responsibility of the attending provider to determine if the patient can be allowed to perform temporary duties with or without restrictions.

Pain relief will likely be a concern during recovery. Pain can be effectively managed with passive and active therapies, nonopioid pain relievers, or short-term opioids. For information and tools on how to use opioids in the perioperative period, see Washington State's L&I's opioid prescribing guideline at www.LNI.opioids.wa.gov.

Evidence shows that work accommodation combined with conservative care during the early recovery period can help prevent disability. Jobsite modifications are dependent on the nature of the patient's work tasks, his or her injury, and his or her response to rehabilitation. Typically, factors such as lifting, pulling, and repetitive overhead work

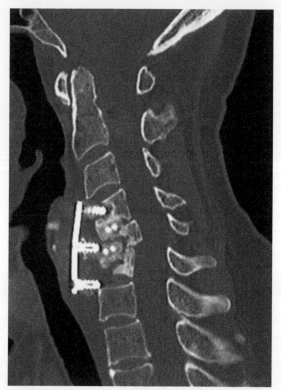

Fig. 12. Sagittal CT image in the same patient demonstrating loosening of the fixation screws and pseudoarthrosis of the interbody grafts.

require modifications in position, force, repetitions, and/or duration. Those workers returning to jobs with heavy lifting or prolonged overhead work may need additional weeks of rehabilitation.

ACKNOWLEDGMENTS

The guideline was largely developed in 2014 by the Washington State Labor and Industries Industrial Insurance Meical Advisory Committee (IIMAC) and its subcommittee on cervical guidelines. Acknowledgments and gratitude go to all subcommittee members, clinical experts, and consultants who contributed to the guideline: B. Lang MD, A. Friedman MD, K. Harmon MD, K. Nilson MD, F. Farrokhi MD, M. Lee MD, JC. Leveque MD, H. Allen MD, J. Babington MD, M. Curatolo MD, K. Reger MD, S. Fowler-Koorn RN, T. Kjerulf MD, K. O'Bara MD, L. Glass MD, H. Stockbridge MD, MPH, N. Reul MD MPH, and G. Franklin MD, MPH.

REFERENCES

1. Todd AG. Cervical spine: degenerative conditions. Curr Rev Musculoskelet Med 2011;4(4):168–74.
2. Kelly JC, Groarke PJ, Butler JS, et al. The natural history and clinical syndromes of degenerative cervical spondylosis. Adv Orthop 2012;2012:393642.

3. Matsumoto M, Fujimura Y, Suzuki N, et al. MRI of cervical intervertebral discs in asymptomatic subjects. J Bone Joint Surg Br 1998;80(1):19–24.

4. Lehto IJ, Tertti MO, Komu ME, et al. Age-related MRI changes at 0.1 T in cervical discs in asymptomatic subjects. Neuroradiology 1994;36(1):49–53.

5. Patil PG, Turner DA, Pietrobon R. National trends in surgical procedures for degenerative cervical spine disease: 1990-2000. Neurosurgery 2005;57(4): 753–8 [discussion: 753–8].

6. Wang MC, Kreuter W, Wolfla CE, et al. Trends and variations in cervical spine surgery in the United States: Medicare beneficiaries, 1992 to 2005. Spine (Phila Pa 1976) 2009;34(9):955–61 [discussion: 962–3].

7. Alosh H, Li D, Riley LH 3rd, et al. Health care burden of anterior cervical spine surgery: national trends in hospital charges and length of stay, 2000 to 2009. J Spinal Disord Tech 2015;28(1):5–11.

8. Buitenhuis J, de Jong PJ, Jaspers JP, et al. Work disability after whiplash: a prospective cohort study. Spine (Phila Pa 1976) 2009;34(3):262–7.

9. Funk JR, Cormier JM, Manoogian SJ. Comparison of risk factors for cervical spine, head, serious, and fatal injury in rollover crashes. Accid Anal Prev 2012; 45:67–74.

10. Fredo HL, Rizvi SA, Lied B, et al. The epidemiology of traumatic cervical spine fractures: a prospective population study from Norway. Scand J Trauma Resusc Emerg Med 2012;20:85.

11. Nelson DW, Martin MJ, Martin ND, et al. Evaluation of the risk of noncontiguous fractures of the spine in blunt trauma. J Trauma Acute Care Surg 2013;75(1):135–9.

12. Schoenfeld AJ, Dunn JC, Bader JO, et al. The nature and extent of war injuries sustained by combat specialty personnel killed and wounded in Afghanistan and Iraq, 2003–2011. J Trauma Acute Care Surg 2013;75(2):287–91.

13. Schoenfeld AJ, Newcomb RL, Pallis MP, et al. Characterization of spinal injuries sustained by American service members killed in Iraq and Afghanistan: a study of 2,089 instances of spine trauma. J Trauma Acute Care Surg 2013;74(4):1112–8.

14. Available at: http://law.justia.com/cases/washington/supreme-court/1987/53022-0-1.html.

15. Jette DU, Jette AM. Physical therapy and health outcomes in patients with spinal impairments. Phys Ther 1996;76(9):930–41 [discussion: 942–5].

16. Saal JS, Saal JA, Yurth EF. Nonoperative management of herniated cervical intervertebral disc with radiculopathy. Spine (Phila Pa 1976) 1996;21(16):1877–83.

17. Kuijper B, Tans JT, Beelen A, et al. Cervical collar or physiotherapy versus wait and see policy for recent onset cervical radiculopathy: randomised trial. BMJ 2009;339:b3883.

18. Anderberg L, Annertz M, Persson L, et al. Transforaminal steroid injections for the treatment of cervical radiculopathy: a prospective and randomised study. Eur Spine J 2007;16(3):321–8.

19. Kolstad F, Leivseth G, Nygaard OP. Transforaminal steroid injections in the treatment of cervical radiculopathy. A prospective outcome study. Acta Neurochir (Wien) 2005;147(10):1065–70 [discussion: 1070].

20. Available at: http://www.fda.gov/downloads/drugs/drugsafety/ucm394286.pdf.

21. Hauerberg J, Kosteljanetz M, Boge-Rasmussen T, et al. Anterior cervical discectomy with or without fusion with ray titanium cage: a prospective randomized clinical study. Spine (Phila Pa 1976) 2008;33(5):458–64.

22. Xie JC, Hurlbert RJ. Discectomy versus discectomy with fusion versus discectomy with fusion and instrumentation: a prospective randomized study. Neurosurgery 2007;61(1):107–16 [discussion: 116–7].

23. Savolainen S, Rinne J, Hernesniemi J. A prospective randomized study of anterior single-level cervical disc operations with long-term follow-up: surgical fusion is unnecessary. Neurosurgery 1998;43(1):51–5.
24. Jagannathan J, Sherman JH, Szabo T, et al. The posterior cervical foraminotomy in the treatment of cervical disc/osteophyte disease: a single-surgeon experience with a minimum of 5 years' clinical and radiographic follow-up. J Neurosurg Spine 2009;10(4):347–56.
25. Fehlings MG, Arvin B. Surgical management of cervical degenerative disease: the evidence related to indications, impact, and outcome. J Neurosurg Spine 2009;11(2):97–100.
26. Clarke MJ, Ecker RD, Krauss WE, et al. Same-segment and adjacent-segment disease following posterior cervical foraminotomy. J Neurosurg Spine 2007; 6(1):5–9.
27. Lawrence BD, Jacobs WB, Norvell DC, et al. Anterior versus posterior approach for treatment of cervical spondylotic myelopathy: a systematic review. Spine (Phila Pa 1976) 2013;38(22 Suppl 1):S173–82.
28. Fehlings MG, Barry S, Kopjar B, et al. Anterior vs posterior surgical approaches to treat cervical spondylotic myelopathy: outcomes of the prospective multicenter AOSpine North America CSM study in 264 patients. Spine (Phila Pa 1976) 2013; 38(26):2247–52.
29. Liu X, Min S, Zhang H, et al. Anterior corpectomy versus posterior laminoplasty for multilevel cervical myelopathy: a systematic review and meta-analysis. Eur Spine J 2014;23(2):362–72.
30. Gao Y, Liu M, Li T, et al. A meta-analysis comparing the results of cervical disc arthroplasty with anterior cervical discectomy and fusion (ACDF) for the treatment of symptomatic cervical disc disease. J Bone Joint Surg Am 2013; 95(6):555–61.
31. Jawahar A, Cavanaugh DA, Kerr EJ 3rd, et al. Total disc arthroplasty does not affect the incidence of adjacent segment degeneration in cervical spine: results of 93 patients in three prospective randomized clinical trials. Spine J 2010;10(12): 1043–8.
32. Coric D, Kim PK, Clemente JD, et al. Prospective randomized study of cervical arthroplasty and anterior cervical discectomy and fusion with long-term follow-up: results in 74 patients from a single site. J Neurosurg Spine 2013;18(1):36–42.
33. Blumenthal SL, Ohnmeiss DD, Guyer RD, et al. Reoperations in cervical total disc replacement compared with anterior cervical fusion: results compiled from multiple prospective food and drug administration investigational device exemption trials conducted at a single site. Spine (Phila Pa 1976) 2013;38(14):1177–82.
34. Heller JG, Sasso RC, Papadopoulos SM, et al. Comparison of BRYAN cervical disc arthroplasty with anterior cervical decompression and fusion: clinical and radiographic results of a randomized, controlled, clinical trial. Spine (Phila Pa 1976) 2009;34(2):101–7.
35. Mummaneni PV, Burkus JK, Haid RW, et al. Clinical and radiographic analysis of cervical disc arthroplasty compared with allograft fusion: a randomized controlled clinical trial. J Neurosurg Spine 2007;6(3):198–209.
36. Zhang X, Chen C, Zhang Y, et al. Randomized, controlled, multicenter, clinical trial comparing BRYAN cervical disc arthroplasty with anterior cervical decompression and fusion in China. Spine (Phila Pa 1976) 2012;37(6):433–8.
37. Sasso RC, Anderson PA, Riew KD, et al. Results of cervical arthroplasty compared with anterior discectomy and fusion: four-year clinical outcomes in a prospective, randomized controlled trial. J Bone Joint Surg Am 2011;93(18):1684–92.

38. Taunt CJ Jr, Sidhu KS, Andrew SA. Somatosensory evoked potential monitoring during anterior cervical discectomy and fusion. Spine (Phila Pa 1976) 2005; 30(17):1970–2.

39. Khan MH, Smith PN, Balzer JR, et al. Intraoperative somatosensory evoked potential monitoring during cervical spine corpectomy surgery: experience with 508 cases. Spine (Phila Pa 1976) 2006;31(4):E105–13.

40. Peeling L, Hentschel S, Fox R, et al. Intraoperative spinal cord and nerve root monitoring: a survey of Canadian spine surgeons. Can J Surg 2010;53(5):324–8.

41. Schwartz DM, Sestokas AK, Dormans JP, et al. Transcranial electric motor evoked potential monitoring during spine surgery: is it safe? Spine (Phila Pa 1976) 2011; 36(13):1046–9.

42. Hilibrand AS, Schwartz DM, Sethuraman V, et al. Comparison of transcranial electric motor and somatosensory evoked potential monitoring during cervical spine surgery. J Bone Joint Surg Am 2004;86-A(6):1248–53.

43. Kim DH, Zaremski J, Kwon B, et al. Risk factors for false positive transcranial motor evoked potential monitoring alerts during surgical treatment of cervical myelopathy. Spine (Phila Pa 1976) 2007;32(26):3041–6.

44. Virginia Mason Medical Center and Group Health Cooperative, Guideline: Intraoperative neurophysiological monitoring (IONM). 2013.

45. Hilibrand AS, Fye MA, Emery SE, et al. Impact of smoking on the outcome of anterior cervical arthrodesis with interbody or strut-grafting. J Bone Joint Surg Am 2001;83-A(5):668–73.

46. Goldberg EJ, Singh K, Van U, et al. Comparing outcomes of anterior cervical discectomy and fusion in workman's versus non-workman's compensation population. Spine J 2002;2(6):408–14.

47. Mok JM, Cloyd JM, Bradford DS, et al. Reoperation after primary fusion for adult spinal deformity: rate, reason, and timing. Spine (Phila Pa 1976) 2009;34(8): 832–9.

48. Kim HJ, Moon SH, Kim HS, et al. Diabetes and smoking as prognostic factors after cervical laminoplasty. J Bone Joint Surg Br 2008;90(11):1468–72.

49. Hilibrand AS, Carlson GD, Palumbo MA, et al. Radiculopathy and myelopathy at segments adjacent to the site of a previous anterior cervical arthrodesis. J Bone Joint Surg Am 1999;81(4):519–28.

50. Lee MJ, Dettori JR, Standaert CJ, et al. The natural history of degeneration of the lumbar and cervical spines: a systematic review. Spine (Phila Pa 1976) 2012; 37(22 Suppl):S18–30.

51. Wilder FV, Fahlman L, Donnelly R. Radiographic cervical spine osteoarthritis progression rates: a longitudinal assessment. Rheumatol Int 2011;31(1):45–8.

52. Acikbas SC, Ermol C, Akyuz M, et al. Assessment of adjacent segment degeneration in and between patients treated with anterior or posterior cervical simple discectomy. Turk Neurosurg 2010;20(3):334–40.

53. Lundine KM, Davis G, Rogers M, et al. Prevalence of adjacent segment disc degeneration in patients undergoing anterior cervical discectomy and fusion based on pre-operative MRI findings. J Clin Neurosci 2014;21(1):82–5.

54. Coric D, Cassis J, Carew JD, et al. Prospective study of cervical arthroplasty in 98 patients involved in 1 of 3 separate investigational device exemption studies from a single investigational site with a minimum 2-year follow-up. Clinical article. J Neurosurg Spine 2010;13(6):715–21.

55. Maldonado CV, Paz RD, Martin CB. Adjacent-level degeneration after cervical disc arthroplasty versus fusion. Eur Spine J 2011;20(Suppl 3):403–7.

56. Nunley PD, Jawahar A, Kerr EJ 3rd, et al. Factors affecting the incidence of symptomatic adjacent-level disease in cervical spine after total disc arthroplasty: 2- to 4-year follow-up of 3 prospective randomized trials. Spine (Phila Pa 1976) 2012;37(6):445–51.
57. Song JS, Choi BW, Song KJ. Risk factors for the development of adjacent segment disease following anterior cervical arthrodesis for degenerative cervical disease: comparison between fusion methods. J Clin Neurosci 2013;21(5): 794–8.
58. Verma K, Gandhi SD, Maltenfort M, et al. Rate of adjacent segment disease in cervical disc arthroplasty versus single-level fusion: meta-analysis of prospective studies. Spine (Phila Pa 1976) 2013;38(26):2253–7.
59. Coric D, Nunley PD, Guyer RD, et al. Prospective, randomized, multicenter study of cervical arthroplasty: 269 patients from the Kineflex|C artificial disc investigational device exemption study with a minimum 2-year follow-up: clinical article. J Neurosurg Spine 2011;15(4):348–58.
60. Burkus JK, Haid RW, Traynelis VC, et al. Long-term clinical and radiographic outcomes of cervical disc replacement with the Prestige disc: results from a prospective randomized controlled clinical trial. J Neurosurg Spine 2010;13(3):308–18.
61. Nabhan A, Steudel WI, Pape D, et al. Segmental kinematics and adjacent level degeneration following disc replacement versus fusion: RCT with three years of follow-up. J Long Term Eff Med Implants 2007;17(3):229–36.
62. Murrey D, Janssen M, Delamarter R, et al. Results of the prospective, randomized, controlled multicenter Food and Drug Administration investigational device exemption study of the ProDisc-C total disc replacement versus anterior discectomy and fusion for the treatment of 1-level symptomatic cervical disc disease. Spine J 2009;9(4):275–86.

Diagnosis and Treatment of Work-Related Ulnar Neuropathy at the Elbow

Gregory T. Carter, MD, MS[a],*, Michael D. Weiss, MD[b],
Andrew S. Friedman, MD[c], Christopher H. Allan, MD[d],
Larry Robinson, MD[e]

KEYWORDS

- Ulnar neuropathy • Ulnar entrapment • Ulnar neuritis • Cubital tunnel syndrome
- Repetitive strain injury

KEY POINTS

- Ulnar neuropathy at the elbow (UNE) is the second most common entrapment neuropathy after carpal tunnel syndrome (CTS). UNE occurs most commonly at the elbow due to mechanical forces that produce traction or ischemia to the nerve.
- Electrodiagnostic (EDX) studies can help to objectively locate, confirm, and quantify the severity of ulnar nerve compression.
- Management should include modification of activities that exacerbate symptoms, nighttime splinting, and/or padding the elbow to prevent direct compression. Surgical treatment should be considered if the condition does not improve despite conservative treatment and the condition interferes with work or activities of daily living.

INTRODUCTION

It is well known that work-related upper limb musculoskeletal disorders, particularly nerve entrapment, remain a difficult and costly problem in industrialized countries. Upper extremity entrapment neuropathies may be misdiagnosed as lateral or medial epicondylitis, de Quervain disease, among many others. Ulnar nerve entrapment occurs most commonly at the elbow due to mechanical forces that produce traction,

[a] St Luke's Rehabilitation Institute, 711 South Cowley Avenue, Spokane, WA 99202, USA;
[b] Department of Neurology, University of Washington School of Medicine, 1959 NE, Pacific Avenue, Seattle, WA 98195, USA; [c] Department of Physical Medicine and Rehabilitation, Neuroscience Institute, Virginia Mason Medical Center, Seattle, WA 98101, USA; [d] Department of Orthopedic Surgery, Hand and Microsurgery Section, Harborview Medical Center, The University of Washington School of Medicine, Seattle, WA 98195, USA; [e] Rehabilitation Services, Physical Medicine and Rehabilitation, Sunnybrook Health Sciences Centre, University of Toronto, Toronto, Ontario M4N 3M5, Canada
* Corresponding author.
E-mail address: gtcarter@uw.edu

Phys Med Rehabil Clin N Am 26 (2015) 513–522
http://dx.doi.org/10.1016/j.pmr.2015.04.002
1047-9651/15/$ – see front matter © 2015 Elsevier Inc. All rights reserved.

pmr.theclinics.com

compression, or ischemia to the ulnar nerve. However, it may be misdiagnosed as CTS, radial tunnel syndrome, and cervicobrachial neuralgia. Despite the high frequency of work-related musculoskeletal disorders, the relation between work conditions and ulnar nerve entrapment at the elbow has not been the object of much research. Predictive factors associated with the onset of ulnar nerve entrapment at the elbow are not yet well delineated. Ulnar nerve entrapment at the elbow is typically associated with biomechanical risk factors (ie, holding a tool in position, repetitively).[1]

For the sake of clarity regarding nomenclature, ulnar neuropathy at the elbow is now considered the preferred term and is used in this article. Terms such as cubital tunnel syndrome or ulnar neuritis are still used by clinicians and may yet be seen in the literature. However, these terms are nonspecific descriptors often used interchangeably for any problem possibly relating to a nerve injury or entrapment near the elbow. After CTS, UNE is the second most common entrapment neuropathy.[1] A differential diagnosis for UNE includes cervical radiculopathy, brachial plexopathy, and compression of the ulnar nerve at the wrist.[1] Potential sites of UNE include Osborne ligament at the cubital tunnel, the arcade of Struthers (particularly after ulnar nerve transposition, when the nerve can be tethered), the medial intermuscular septum, the medial epicondyle, the flexor-pronator aponeurosis, and rarely an accessory muscle, the anconeus epitrochlearis.[2] Entrapment may also occur from soft-tissue structures such as tumors or ganglions, bony abnormalities due to fractures, osteophytes (bone spurs), or subluxation of the ulnar nerve over the medial epicondyle with elbow flexion. A tardy ulnar nerve palsy may be seen in association deformities of the elbow secondary to a supracondylar fracture of the humerus. This condition may occur when the ulnar nerve becomes entrapped by scar tissue, which may produce anterior displacement of the nerve with elbow flexion, which may then spontaneously reduce back into the ulnar nerve groove with elbow extension.[3] In general, work-relatedness and appropriate symptoms and objective signs must be present to establish a legitimate claim. EDX studies, including nerve conduction velocity (NCV) studies and needle electromyography (EMG), should be scheduled immediately to corroborate the clinical diagnosis.

ESTABLISHING WORK-RELATEDNESS

Work-related activities may also cause or contribute to the development of UNE. Establishing work-relatedness requires all of the following:

1. Exposure: Workplace activities that contribute to or cause UNE
2. Outcome: A diagnosis of UNE that meets the diagnostic criteria given in section Making The Diagnosis
3. Relationship: Generally accepted scientific evidence, which establishes on a more probable than not basis (greater than 50%) that the workplace activities (exposure) in an individual case contributed to the development or worsening of the condition (outcome)

Although the exact incidence and prevalence are uncertain, UNE is second only to CTS as the most common peripheral nerve entrapment. From 1995 to 2000, approximately 2800 claims for work-related UNE were reported to the Washington State Department of Labor and Industries.[4] Approximately one-quarter of these patients received surgical treatment, whereas the remainder was treated conservatively. Time loss payments were paid to 93% of the surgery group and 61% of the conservatively treated group.

Certain work-related activities have been associated with UNE, such as activities requiring repetitive or sudden elbow flexion or extension, intensive use of hand tools, or repeated trauma or pressure to the elbow.[1,5,6] Jobs in which these activities occur may include but are not limited to the following: repetitive lifting, leaning on elbows at desk or work bench, working in tight places, shoveling, digging, hammering, using hand saws or large power machinery, and operating boring and punching machines. Several specific occupations have been associated with UNE,[1,3,4] including carpenter, painter, glass cutter, musician, seamstress, packaging worker, assembly line worker, shoe and clothing industry worker, and food industry worker. This list is not exhaustive and is meant only as a guide in the consideration of work-relatedness.

Both high body mass index (BMI) and low BMI have been reported as risk factors for UNE.[7] Landau and colleagues[7] retrospectively analyzed the EDX records of subjects with UNE. The BMI was calculated for 50 patients with a sole diagnosis of UNE and compared with the BMI of 50 patients with CTS and 50 control subjects. The difference in BMI between patients with UNE and normal patients was significant (P<.01). In the control groups, increasing BMI directly correlated with increasing ulnar motor NCV across the elbow but not with forearm NCV. The results suggested that across-elbow (AE) ulnar motor NCV may be falsely increased in patients with a high BMI, probably because of distance measurement factors. Slender individuals seem to have comparatively slower AE ulnar NCVs and may also be at increased risk for developing UNE.

MAKING THE DIAGNOSIS

For the purposes of this article, the case definition of confirmed UNE includes appropriate symptoms, objective physical findings (signs), and abnormal results on EDX studies. A provisional diagnosis of UNE may be made based on appropriate symptoms and objective signs, but confirmation of the diagnosis requires abnormal results on EDX studies. The anatomy of the ulnar nerve and areas of entrapment are illustrated in **Fig. 1**.

Symptoms and Signs

The primary symptom associated with UNE is diminished sensation or dysesthesias in the ring and small fingers (fourth and fifth digits), often coupled with pain in the proximal medial aspect of the elbow.[6] Motor symptoms may include progressive weakness, with inability to separate fingers, loss of power grip, and poor dexterity. Nonspecific symptoms (eg, pain without sensory loss, "dropping things") by themselves are not diagnostic of UNE. Symptoms of UNE may worsen at night. Symptom provocation has been described with Tinel sign (tapping over the cubital tunnel) or by sustained (60 seconds) elbow flexion with or without manual compression of the ulnar nerve at or proximal to the cubital tunnel.[8] Alone, these findings are neither sensitive nor specific for the diagnosis of UNE.

Objective findings on physical examination should be localized to muscles supplied by the ulnar nerve or sensory impairment in an ulnar distribution. In the forearm, the muscular branch of the ulnar nerve innervates the flexor carpi ulnaris and the flexor digitorum profundus (medial half). In the hand, the deep branch of the ulnar nerve innervates the hypothenar muscles (opponens digiti minimi, abductor digiti minimi [ADM], flexor digiti minimi brevis), the adductor pollicis, the flexor pollicis brevis (deep head), the third and fourth lumbrical muscles, and the dorsal and palmar interossei. In the hand, the superficial branch of the ulnar nerve innervates the palmaris brevis.

Weakness of the hand intrinsic muscles may be tested by looking for a positive Froment sign, which is a contraction of flexor pollicis longus to compensate for a weak adductor pollicis.[5] Testing involves having the patient attempt to hold a flat object (ie, a piece of paper) between the index finger and thumb. The examiner then tries

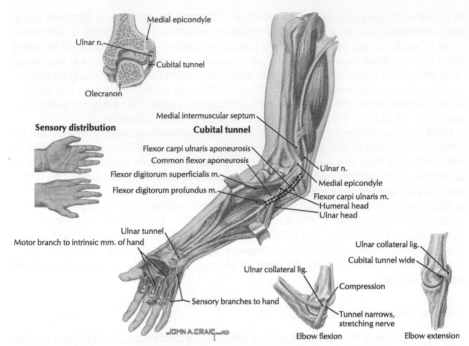

Fig. 1. The anatomy of the ulnar nerve and areas of entrapment. Copyright © 2015 Elsevier Inc. All rights reserved. www.netterimages.com.

to pull the object out of the patient's hands. A normal individual is able to maintain a hold on the object without difficulty. Because of weakness in the ulnar nerve–innervated adductor pollicis muscle, a patient with an ulnar nerve lesion has difficulty maintaining a hold on the object and compensates by contracting the flexor pollicis longus muscle to achieve a grip.

In more advanced cases, intrinsic muscle atrophy becomes visibly evident (eg, first dorsal interosseous [FDI]). In severe cases, hand opening reveals a characteristic ulnar claw posture, with hyperextension of the metacaropophalangeal joints and flexion of the interphalangeal joints.[2] This posture should not be confused with the median neuropathy benediction sign seen with hand closing. Ulnar sensory impairment can be demonstrated using Semmes-Weinstein monofilaments and should be localized to the ulnar side of the ring finger and the small finger and ulnar aspect of the hand. There seems to be a high frequency of diagnostic imprecision for cases handled within the workers' compensation system. In the general population, UNE typically occurs as an isolated mononeuropathy, with coincidence of UNE and CTS being uncommon. However, in the workman compensation setting, approximately 60% of UNE surgical patients have a concomitant diagnosis of CTS, usually made before a diagnosis of UNE.[4] Every effort should be made to objectively verify the diagnosis of UNE before considering surgery.

ELECTRODIAGNOSTIC STUDIES
Nerve Conduction Studies

EDX studies, including both nerve conduction studies (NCSs) and needle EMG, can help to objectively locate, confirm, and quantify the severity of ulnar nerve compression.[9–13] The ulnar nerve–innervated muscles are given in **Box 1**.

> **Box 1**
> **Ulnar nerve–innervated muscles**
>
> *Forearm*
>
> - Flexor carpi ulnaris
> - Flexor digitorum profundus (medial half)
>
> *Hand*
>
> - Hypothenar muscles: opponens digiti minimi; abductor digiti minimi; flexor digiti minimi brevis
> - Adductor pollicis
> - Flexor pollicis brevis deep head
> - Lumbrical muscles (third and fourth)
> - Dorsal interossei
> - Palmar interossei
> - Palmaris brevis (via the superficial branch of the ulnar nerve)

There remains some debate regarding how best to use ulnar motor nerve conduction velocity (MNCV) to identify UNE. NCVs measured across the elbow with the ulnar nerve–innervated hand intrinsic musculature (abductor digiti minimi or first dorsal interosseus muscles) are used for motor conduction velocity determination, with the elbow held with a moderate degree of flexion (70°–90°).[11]

Shakir and colleagues[9] used receiver operator characteristic (ROC) curves to compare absolute AE MNCV with MNCV difference between elbow and forearm segments, with recording from ADM and FDI muscles. With 95% specificity, the sensitivities of AE MNCV were considerably better than studying the MNCV difference between elbow and forearm segments (80% at ADM, 77% at FDI). The ROC curves showed MNCV to be superior across all amplitude subgroups, although confidence intervals did overlap when the amplitude of responses was high. Recording from both FDI and ADM may increase sensitivity.

Early studies by Maynard and Stolov[10] indicated that the experimental error in calculating NCV is influenced by errors of latency and distance measurements. Their original data implied that a minimum distance of 10 cm should be used when calculating NCV because of an increase in error of 25% or more at shorter distances. However, studies using modern EDX equipment show that NCV can reasonably be calculated at distances less than 10 cm, perhaps as low as 5 to 6 cm.[11–13]

There must be evidence of ulnar nerve demyelination with or without axon loss to confirm a diagnosis of UNE and should include at least 2 of the following motor nerve conduction abnormalities:

1. Slowing of AE to below elbow (BE) NCV to less than 50 m/s in either the ADM or FDI
2. Focal slowing on inching studies of the ulnar nerve across the elbow, defined as a latency difference exceeding 0.7 milliseconds across a 2-cm segment (or 0.4 milliseconds across a 1-cm segment)
3. Compound muscle action potential (CMAP) amplitude decrease of greater than 20% between AE and BE waveforms (for findings 3 and 4, and particularly when there is an amplitude drop between wrist and BE, the presence of a Martin-Gruber anastomosis must be excluded)

4. CMAP duration increase of greater than 30% between AE and BE waveforms (for findings 3 and 4, and particularly when there is an amplitude drop between wrist and BE, the presence of a Martin-Gruber anastomosis must be excluded)

To exclude the presence of polyneuropathy as a cause of the abnormalities described earlier, evaluation of another motor and sensory nerve must be normal. Given that most neuropathies are sensory predominant, checking another sensory nerve is just as critical as checking another motor nerve. Ulnar sensory EDX abnormalities alone are considered to be nonspecific and nonlocalizing and hence cannot alone be used to confirm a diagnosis of UNE. There is also not sufficient reference data at this point to support using sensory studies to confirm the diagnosis of UNE. With respect to prognosis, there is some evidence that large compound muscle action potentials elicited by distal stimulation and presence of conduction block are associated with a good prognosis.[14]

Needle Electromyography

EMG studies are usually normal if the NCSs are entirely normal and there are no atypical or unexplained signs or symptoms. Isolated needle EMG findings in the setting of normal NCSs are typically not seen in UNE and could indicate another diagnosis. If there are clinical findings suggesting a diagnosis other than or in addition to UNE, needle EMG may be appropriate, for example, to evaluate the following:

1. Possible median neuropathy, demonstrated by clinical weakness or atrophy of the thenar muscles, or abnormal median NCS
2. Possible peripheral polyneuropathy, such as from diabetes
3. Possible traumatic nerve injury following acute trauma to the distal upper extremity
4. Possible cervical radiculopathy, with neck stiffness and radiating pain

Needle EMG study is not considered sufficient to establish a diagnosis of ulnar neuropathy in the absence of nerve conduction changes. If EMG is performed, the most helpful needle EMG finding in ulnar neuropathy is abnormal rest activity in the form of fibrillation potentials and positive sharp waves in ulnar nerve–innervated muscles in the hand and forearm, which could suggest ongoing axonal injury.

OTHER DIAGNOSTIC TESTS

Some studies have demonstrated that MRI neurography and ultrasonography (US) have promise in the diagnosis of UNE.[15–18] However, the clinical utility of these tests has not yet been proven. Although these tests may be useful in unusual circumstances in which NCV results are normal but there are appropriate clinical symptoms, at this time the use of these tests should be considered investigational and used only in a research setting. A meta-analysis of the literature for US in the diagnosis of UNE revealed 14 clinical trials, 7 of which were suitable for further analysis. The measurement of ulnar nerve size by US shows reasonable accuracy. The most commonly noted abnormality in patients with UNE was an increased cross-sectional area of the ulnar nerve at the elbow. However, the investigators noted that many studies had methodological flaws, including that there is tremendous variability in US techniques.[15] A recent study evaluated sensitivity and specificity of US and EDX studies in 30 patients with UNE and 33 controls.[18] EDX studies were used as the gold standard for diagnosis and had a sensitivity for UNE of 63.3% and a specificity of 87.9%. US had a sensitivity of 76.7% and a specificity of 72.7%. This pilot study indicates that US may be slightly more sensitive if complaints exist for 6 months or less. However, if complaints persisted for more than 6 months, sensitivity and specificity of the

EDX studies were superior.[18] Thus, the role of US in UNE seems promising but is not yet clearly established and more prospective studies are needed.

TREATMENT
Conservative Treatment

Treatment may be conservative or surgical, but optimal management remains controversial. Nonsurgical therapy may be considered in cases in which a provisional diagnosis has been made (ie, it has not been confirmed by EDX testing). Surgical treatment should be provided only in cases in which the diagnosis of UNE has been confirmed by abnormal EDX studies, as the potential benefits of UNE surgery outweigh the risks of surgery only when the diagnosis of UNE has been confirmed by abnormal results on EDX studies. Conservative treatment is reasonable for patients presenting with early or mild symptoms, for example, intermittent dysesthesias, minimal motor findings, and normal results on EDX testing. The goals of conservative treatment are to reduce the frequency and severity of symptoms and to prevent further progression of the condition.[3,19] Management should include modification of activities that exacerbate symptoms, night-time splinting, or padding the elbow to prevent direct compression. Splinting has been reported to provide improvement within 1 month for some patients.[20,21] However, there is no consensus on the duration of conservative treatment, and the recommended length of time varies between 1 month and 1 year. Patients do not usually need time off from work activities before surgery unless they present with objective weakness in the distribution of the ulnar nerve that compromises workplace safety or limits work activities.

Surgical Treatment

Optimal surgical management of cubital tunnel syndrome remains uncertain despite the publication of numerous case series, observational studies, systematic reviews, and, in recent years, some randomized controlled studies. Surgical treatment should be considered if the condition does not improve despite conservative treatment and interferes with work or activities of daily living. Surgery should include exploration of the ulnar nerve throughout its course around the elbow and release of all compressive structures.[22,23] Complete release may require nerve decompression at multiple sites and may also require Z-lengthening of the flexor pronator origin, if elevated to allow for anterior submuscular transposition. A Cochrane review analyzed the available literature regarding the effectiveness and safety of conservative and surgical treatments in UNE.[24] The review included only randomized controlled clinical trials (RCTs) or quasi-RCTs evaluating people with clinical symptoms suggesting the presence of UNE. The results identified 6 RCTs (430 participants), with moderate quality evidence, for inclusion in the review. Two meta-analyses evaluated 3 clinical trials with 261 participants as well as 2 neurophysiologic studies with 101 participants. Outcomes of simple decompression versus decompression with submuscular or subcutaneous transposition were compared. No differences in outcome were identified between simple decompression and transposition of the ulnar nerve for both clinical and neurophysiologic improvement. Providing patients with information on avoiding prolonged movements or positions seemed to be effective in improving subjective discomfort. Night splinting and nerve gliding exercises in addition to the information did not produce further improvement. The investigators concluded that the available evidence is not sufficient to identify the best treatment of idiopathic UNE based on clinical, neurophysiologic, and imaging characteristics. The results of this meta-analysis suggest that simple decompression and decompression with transposition are equally effective in idiopathic UNE, including when the nerve impairment is severe. In mild cases, evidence from 1 small RCT of conservative treatment showed that information on movements or positions to avoid may reduce subjective discomfort. These results may not be reflective of a work-related UNE.

The indications for surgical intervention in the setting of UNE are not as clear cut as with the more commonly encountered CTS. In CTS, there is a much more predictable progression of the pathophysiology and the cause among cases is much more similar. In ulnar neuropathy, the pathophysiology may be wide ranging, very different, and variable. Some forms of UNE have pathophysiology that is predominantly axonal, whereas other forms are more demyelinating. There are also many unanswered questions, including whether or not a surgically transposed ulnar nerve actually heals faster after a singular injury as opposed to a chronically entrapped nerve; this has led to considerable variability in outcomes.[25–27]

Return to Work

Timeliness of the diagnosis can be a critical factor influencing return to work (RTW). Among workers with upper extremity disorders, 7% of workers account for 75% of the long-term disability.[28] A large prospective study in the Washington State workers' compensation system identified several important predictors of long-term disability: low expectations of RTW, no offer of a job accommodation, and high physical demands on the job.[29] Identifying and attending to these risk factors when patients have not returned to work within 2 to 3 weeks of the initial clinical presentation may improve their chances of RTW. Washington State workers diagnosed accurately and early were far more likely to RTW than workers whose conditions were diagnosed weeks or months later. Early coordination of care with improved timeliness and effective communication with the workplace is also likely to help prevent long-term disability. How soon a patient can RTW depends on the type of surgery performed and when rehabilitation begins. Most patients requiring a UNE release alone can return to light duty work within 3 weeks.

REFERENCES

1. Descatha A, Leclerc A, Chastang JF, et al, Study Group on Repetitive Work. Incidence of ulnar nerve entrapment at the elbow in repetitive work. Scand J Work Environ Health 2004;30(3):234–40.
2. Husain SN, Kaufmann RA. The diagnosis and treatment of cubital tunnel syndrome. Curr Orthop Pract 2008;19(5):470–4.
3. Szabo RM, Kwak C. Natural history and conservative management of cubital tunnel syndrome. Hand Clin 2007;23:311–8.
4. Burns PB, Kim HM, Gaston RG, et al. Predictors of functional outcomes after simple decompression for ulnar neuropathy at the elbow: a multicenter study by the SUN study group. Arch Phys Med Rehabil 2014;95(4):680–5.
5. Piligian G, Herbert R, Hearnes M, et al. Evaluation and management of chronic work-related musculoskeletal disorders of the distal upper extremity. Am J Ind Med 2000;37:75–93.
6. Mondelli M, Grippo A, Mariani M, et al. Carpal tunnel syndrome and ulnar neuropathy at the elbow in floor cleaners. Neurophysiol Clin 2006;36:245–53.
7. Landau ME, Barner KC, Campbell WW. Effect of body mass index on ulnar nerve conduction velocity, ulnar neuropathy at the elbow, and carpal tunnel syndrome. Muscle Nerve 2005;32(3):360–3.

8. Novak CB, Lee GW, Mackinnon SE, et al. Provocative testing for cubital tunnel syndrome. J Hand Surg Am 1994;19:817–20.
9. Shakir A, Micklesen PJ, Robinson LR. Which motor nerve conduction study is best in ulnar neuropathy at the elbow? Muscle Nerve 2004;29(4):585–90.
10. Maynard FM, Stolov WC. Experimental error in determination of nerve conduction velocity. Arch Phys Med Rehabil 1972;53(8):362–72.
11. Landau ME, Barner KC, Campbell WW. Optimal screening distance for ulnar neuropathy at the elbow. Muscle Nerve 2003;27(5):570–4.
12. Landau ME, Diaz MI, Barner KC, et al. Optimal distance for segmental nerve conduction studies revisited. Muscle Nerve 2003;27(3):367–9.
13. Campbell WW. Guidelines in electrodiagnostic medicine. Practice parameter for electrodiagnostic studies in ulnar neuropathy at the elbow. Muscle Nerve Suppl 1999;8:S171–205.
14. Friedrich JM, Robinson LR. Prognostic indicators from electrodiagnostic studies for ulnar neuropathy at the elbow. Muscle Nerve 2011;43(4):596–600.
15. Beekman R, Visser LH, Verhagen WI. Ultrasonography in ulnar neuropathy at the elbow: a critical review. Muscle Nerve 2011;43(5):627–35.
16. van Veen KE, Wesstein M, van Kasteel V. Ultrasonography and electrodiagnostic studies in ulnar neuropathy: an examination of the sensitivity and specificity and the correlations between both diagnostic tools. J Clin Neurophysiol 2014. [Epub ahead of print].
17. Ayromlou H, Tarzamni MK, Daghighi MH, et al. Diagnostic value of ultrasonography and magnetic resonance imaging in ulnar neuropathy at the elbow. ISRN Neurol 2012;2012:491892.
18. Volpe A, Rossato G, Bottanelli M, et al. Ultrasound evaluation of ulnar neuropathy at the elbow: correlation with electrophysiological studies. Rheumatology (Oxford) 2009;48(9):1098–101.
19. Smith T, Nielsen KD, Poulsgaard L. Ulnar neuropathy at the elbow: clinical and electrophysiological outcome of surgical and conservative treatment. Scand J Plast Reconstr Surg Hand Surg 2000;34(2):145–8.
20. Dellon AL, Hament W, Gittelshon A. Nonoperative management of cubital tunnel syndrome: an 8-year prospective study. Neurology 1993;43:1673–7.
21. Hong C, Long H, Kanakamedala RV, et al. Splinting and local steroid injection for the treatment of ulnar neuropathy at the elbow: clinical and electrophysiological examination. Arch Phys Med Rehabil 1996;77:573–7.
22. Song JW, Waljee JF, Burns PB, et al, Surgery for the Ulnar Nerve (SUN) Study Group. An outcome study for ulnar neuropathy at the elbow: a multicenter study by the Surgery for Ulnar Nerve (SUN) study group. Neurosurgery 2013;72(6): 971–81.
23. Giladi AM, Gaston RG, Haase SC, et al, Surgery of the Ulnar Nerve Study Group. Trend of recovery after simple decompression for treatment of ulnar neuropathy at the elbow. Plast Reconstr Surg 2013;131(4):563e–73e.
24. Caliandro P, La Torre G, Padua R, et al. Treatment for ulnar neuropathy at the elbow. Cochrane Database Syst Rev 2012;(7):CD006839.
25. Macadam SA, Gandhi R, Bezuhly M, et al. Simple decompression versus anterior subcutaneous and submuscular transposition of the ulnar nerve for cubital tunnel syndrome: a meta-analysis. J Hand Surg Am 2008;33(8): 1314.e1–12.
26. Blonna D, O'Driscoll SW. Delayed-onset ulnar neuritis after release of elbow contracture: preventive strategies derived from a study of 563 cases. Arthroscopy 2014;30(8):947–56.

27. Martin KD, Dützmann S, Sobottka SB, et al. Retractor-endoscopic nerve decompression in carpal and cubital tunnel syndromes: outcomes in a small series. World Neurosurg 2014;82(1–2):e361–70.
28. Hashemi L, Webster BS, Clance EA, et al. Length of disability and cost of work-related musculoskeletal disorders of the upper extremity. J Occup Environ Med 1998;40:261–9.
29. Turner JA, Franklin G, Fulton-Kehoe D. Early predictors of chronic work disability associated with carpal tunnel syndrome: a longitudinal workers' compensation cohort study. Am J Ind Med 2007;50:489–500.

Work-Related Carpal Tunnel Syndrome
Diagnosis and Treatment Guideline

Gary M. Franklin, MD, MPH[a],*, Andrew S. Friedman, MD[b]

KEYWORDS

- Carpal tunnel syndrome • Causation • Diagnosis • Electrodiagnostic studies
- Evidence-based review • Treatment • Workers' compensation

KEY POINTS

- Carpal tunnel syndrome (CTS) is the most common entrapment neuropathy, and it is associated with a large disease burden in workers' compensation systems.
- The diagnosis in workers' compensation systems should depend on the presence of specific symptoms, signs, and abnormal results of nerve conduction tests consistent with a case definition for the presence of CTS.
- Strong evidence associates the occurrence of CTS with forceful, angular, and repetitive hand use, or with vibration; CTS is less likely to occur in typists or data entry operators but may occur with intensive computer use of at least 12 to 20 h/wk.
- Conservative management in the workers' compensation system should be effective enough to maintain employment; surgical decompression is highly effective and should be entertained in workers who cannot remain at work with conservative management. Patients should continue to work until decompression is undertaken.

INTRODUCTION

CTS is the most commonly diagnosed entrapment neuropathy,[1] and it is associated with a large disease burden in the workers' compensation system.[2–4] The annual incidence in the general population has been reported to be approximately 1 in 1000.[5] The incidence of CTS in Washington (WA) workers' compensation population peaked at approximately 2.73 per 1000 in the mid-1990s.[6] One study estimated 4 to 10 million cases of CTS in the United States in 2005[7]; in 2010, 5 million workers were estimated to have CTS.[8] Among commonly performed ambulatory surgical procedures of the upper extremity, CTS release was twice as frequently as rotator cuff repair (**Table 1**).[9]

[a] Departments of Environmental and Occupational Health Sciences, Neurology, and Health Services, University of Washington, 130 Nickerson, Seattle, WA 98109, USA; [b] Department of Physical Medicine and Rehabilitation, Virginia Mason Medical Center, Seattle, WA 98101, USA
* Corresponding author.
E-mail address: meddir@uw.edu

Phys Med Rehabil Clin N Am 26 (2015) 523–537
http://dx.doi.org/10.1016/j.pmr.2015.04.003
1047-9651/15/$ – see front matter © 2015 Elsevier Inc. All rights reserved.

Table 1		
National estimates of upper extremity ambulatory surgery procedures, 2006		
Procedure	Number of Procedures	Rate/10, 000 Among Those Aged 45–64 y
Carpal tunnel release	576,924	37.3
Rotator cuff repair	272,148	21.1
Shoulder arthroscopy	257,541	17.1

Adapted from Jain NB, Higgins LD, Losina E, et al. Epidemiology of musculoskeletal upper extremity ambulatory surgery in the United States. BMC Musculoskelet Disord 2014;15:4; with permission.

The highest prevalence of CTS procedures in this study, reflecting a much higher rate among women and in people aged 45 to 64 years, also likely reflects similar representations of case demographics in workers' compensation systems.[10]

ESTABLISHING WORK RELATEDNESS

CTS may result from numerous conditions, including inflammatory or noninflammatory arthropathies, recent or remote wrist trauma or fractures, diabetes mellitus, obesity, hypothyroidism, pregnancy, and genetic factors.[6,11,12]

Risk for CTS strongly increases with age and among perimenopausal women for unclear reasons. In the unusual instance that CTS is acutely, traumatically induced, for example, a patient has both CTS and concomitant trauma (fracture or dislocation), the patient may require prompt carpal tunnel release (CTR).

Work-related activities may also cause or contribute to the development of CTS. To establish a diagnosis of work-related CTS, all of the following are required:

1. Exposure: workplace activities that contribute to or cause CTS
2. Outcome: a diagnosis of CTS that meets the diagnostic criteria under "Making the Diagnosis"
3. Relationship: generally accepted scientific evidence, which establishes on a more probable than not basis (greater than 50%) that the workplace activities (exposure) in an individual case contributed to the development or worsening of the condition (outcome).

Several recent meta-analyses and studies have summarized the now well-known risks of work-related CTS involving activities requiring extensive, forceful, repetitive, or prolonged use of the hands and wrists, or exposure to vibration, particularly if these potential risk factors are present in combination (eg, force and repetition or force and posture).[13–15] The risks associated with computer, keyboard, or mouse use are most likely to be present only with long durations of exposure or at least 12 to 20 h/wk of intensive exposure.[16–18] Negative studies have generally not measured exposures at this level of detail.[19–21]

Usually, one or more of the following work conditions occurring on a regular basis could support work relatedness:

1. Forceful use, particularly if repeated
2. Repetitive hand use combined with some element of force, especially for prolonged periods
3. Constant firm gripping of objects
4. Moving or using the hand and wrist against resistance or with force
5. Exposing the hand and wrist to strong regular vibrations
6. Intensive computer, keyboard, or mouse use of at least 12 to 20 h/wk

The types of jobs most mentioned in the literature or reported in the WA workers' compensation data as being associated with CTS are listed in **Table 2**. This list is not an exhaustive one and is meant only to be a guide in the consideration of work relatedness.

MAKING THE DIAGNOSIS
Symptoms and Signs

A case definition for the presence or absence of CTS requires both appropriate symptoms and abnormal nerve conduction velocity (NCV) tests for the diagnosis.[22] Appropriate symptoms include numbness, tingling, or burning pain in the volar aspects of one or both hands, especially noted after work or at night. Nocturnal symptoms are prominent in 50% to 70% of patients. Patients frequently awaken at night or early morning and shake their hands to relieve these symptoms. These symptoms may be reported to be involving the entire hand or be localized to the thumb and first 2 or 3 fingers. A hand pain diagram has been validated for use in localizing sensory symptoms of CTS (appended to the end of this guideline).[23]

If the nerve symptoms are prominent only in the fourth and fifth fingers, a different diagnosis (eg, ulnar neuropathy or C8 radiculopathy) should be considered. Although burning pain is often prominent in the hands and palm side of the wrists, an aching pain may radiate to the medial elbow region or more proximally to the shoulder. Proximal symptoms, especially tingling in the radial part of the hand, combined with lateral elbow pain should raise questions about a possible C6 radiculopathy.

Signs present on physical examination are frequently absent or nonspecific. Hoffmann-Tinel sign (paresthesias radiating in a median nerve distribution with tapping on the wrist or over the median nerve) and Phalen sign (paresthesias radiating in a median nerve distribution within 60 seconds of sustained flexion of the wrist) are frequently described but by themselves are not sensitive or specific for the diagnosis of CTS.[22] The presence of these signs may corroborate the presence of other clear neurologic symptoms. Likewise, nonspecific symptoms, (eg, pain without numbness, tingling, or burning; dropping things) by themselves are not diagnostic of CTS. Signs that occur as CTS becomes more severe include decreased sensation to pin or light touch in the first 3 digits or weakness or atrophy of the muscles of the thenar eminence (especially the abductor pollicis brevis). Unlike Tinel or Phalen signs, the presence of thenar atrophy or weakness may suggest more acute or advanced nerve injury and perhaps the need for more aggressive treatment.

Table 2
Work exposures and the probability of work relatedness

Exposure	Examples of Types of Jobs	Probability of Work Relatedness
Combinations of high force with high repetition and awkward posture, regular strong vibrations	Seafood, fruit, or meat processing or canning; carpentry; roofing; drywall installation; boat building; book binding	High, relative risk >4
Medium to high force, high repetition, or awkward posture alone, on a nearly continuous basis	Dental hygienists, wood products production	Medium, relative risk 2–4
Low force or medium to low repetition alone, on an intermittent basis	Computer or keyboard use	Low, relative risk <2

Every effort should be made to objectively verify the diagnosis of CTS before considering surgery. Although some evidence is conflicted, it has been suggested that patients who have undergone carpal tunnel surgery with normal or near-normal presurgical nerve conduction test results have poorer outcomes than those with electrodiagnostic evidence of median nerve entrapment across the carpal tunnel.[24,25] In rare cases, a steroid injection can be administered into the carpal canal as a therapeutic and diagnostic challenge test. Patients noting a dramatic improvement in symptoms for weeks or months after the injection, but then having recurrence of symptoms, may be considered candidates for surgical CTR. Patients with a negative response may be referred to an appropriate specialist (eg, neurologist, orthopedist, or physiatrist) for further diagnostic evaluation if warranted or be followed up for a 12-month period to monitor for neurologic findings that may develop.

If CTS is not documented by clinical criteria and NCV testing, other clinical problems potentially related to work exposures (eg, tendonitis), should be investigated and treated appropriately. It would also be important to rule out other neurologic causes of tingling in the hands. Referral to an appropriate specialist (neurologist, physiatrist) would be prudent in such cases.

CTS is a common physiologic condition in pregnancy[11]; this is theorized to be due to increased plasma volume and fluid retention that raise the pressure within the carpal tunnel. The symptoms of CTS often improve after childbirth. If they do not, other causes should be pursued.

Electrodiagnostic Studies

Nerve conduction velocity

An easy-to-use worksheet for interpreting electrodiagnostic studies is available at the end of this guideline. The worksheet should be used only when the main purpose of the study is to evaluate a patient for CTS. It is critical to conduct NCV testing in the following situation:

1. The diagnosis of CTS is being considered
2. Patient is on time loss for more than 2 weeks
3. Carpal tunnel decompression surgery is requested

Conceptually, validation of the clinical diagnosis of CTS depends on the finding of slowing of sensory and/or motor fibers of the median nerve across the carpal tunnel. The nerve conduction study methods used to test for slowing should not be affected by temperature (either the temperature should be maintained over 32°C or tests that are not influenced by temperature should be used). These electrodiagnostic studies (EDS) should have a high specificity, good sensitivity, and high degree of reliability. Such tests should also minimize the possibility of age or polyneuropathy creating a misleading or false-positive result; this can often be accomplished by comparing the median nerve to another nerve across the same distance across the wrist.

NCV tests are highly sensitive and specific for CTS.[22] If the patient has a positive clinical picture of CTS but the NCV results are negative, the physician should investigate other competing clinical diagnoses such as pronator syndrome, cervical radiculopathy, or tendonitis. Less than 10% of patients with clinical CTS have normal NCV results.[26–30] In these cases, the treating physician should be sure that the most sensitive and specific NCV tests are done. If not, a request for these tests should be made. In some cases of suspected CTS, the NCV tests can be repeated. However, unless there is a significant intervening event or a substantial change in the clinical assessment, there should be a delay of at least 1 year before repeating the NCV test, because it is unlikely that a difference will be seen at a shorter time interval.

NCV techniques along with their reference values and their upper limits of normal cut points used to corroborate a diagnosis of CTS include the following:

Median motor distal latency (8 cm)
> Note: If median motor distal latency is abnormal, then ulnar motor distal latency at 8 cm must be within normal limits ($\leq$3.9 ms)
> Less than 4.5 ms[9]

Median sensory distal latency 8 cm recorded (palm to wrist) *or* 14 cm recorded (index, long, or ring finger to wrist)
> If either of these tests is used alone, at least one other sensory nerve in the ipsilateral hand should be normal
> Less than 8 cm[10]
> Less than 14 cm

Median − ulnar motor latency difference (abductor pollicis brevis [APB] vs abductor digiti minimi [ADM]) (8 cm)
> Less than 1.6 ms[11]

Median − ulnar sensory latency difference to digits (14 cm), index or long finger compared to ulnar recorded at the small finger, or median − ulnar difference recorded at the ring finger
> Less than 0.5 ms

Median − ulnar sensory latency difference across the palm (8 cm)
> Less than 0.3 ms

Median − radial sensory latency difference to the thumb (10 cm)
> Less than 0.6 ms[12]

Combined sensory index (CSI)
> The CSI is calculated by adding the 3 latency differences[31,32] above: CSI = (median latency at 14 cm − ulnar latency at 14 cm) + (median latency at 8 cm across palm − ulnar latency at 8 cm across palm) + (median latency to thumb at 10 cm − radial latency to thumb at 10 cm)[13,14]
> Less than 0.9 ms

These upper limit cut points are derived from published literature. The limits for sensory latencies are chosen for high specificity (ie, few false-positives).

In all cases, and particularly in cases with borderline NCV results, control for skin temperature should be documented. In general, the above-referenced values hold for skin temperature in the range of 30°C to 34°C. Lower temperatures are associated with falsely slowed NCV results.

The department's (Washington Department of Labor and Industries) policy on EDS follows that of the American Association of Neuromuscular and Electrodiagnostic Medicine. The department does not cover portable NCV tests.

Needle electromyography

Needle electromyography (EMG) sometimes has a role in the electrodiagnostic evaluation of CTS. If the clinical presentation is classic for CTS symptoms and no other signs and/or symptoms, and the result of nerve conduction study is entirely normal, no needle EMG or only limited EMG studies are acceptable. However, there are circumstances in which it would be reasonable to do needle EMG during an evaluation of CTS:

1. Results of nerve conduction studies are abnormal in a manner indicating CTS and the patient demonstrates wasting or clinical weakness of the thenar muscles, or the median motor nerve conduction study is significantly abnormal
2. The electromyographer suspects another possible diagnosis or a neuropathic process other than, or in addition to, CTS (eg, diabetes)

3. There is a history of an acute crush injury or other major trauma to the distal upper extremity
4. There are proximal symptoms (eg, neck stiffness, radiating pain) that suggest cervical radiculopathy may be present.

Quantitative sensory testing

The department does not cover quantitative sensory tests. Several tests of sensory function (vibration, temperature, pressure) have been reported in the scientific literature to be useful in investigational settings to differentiate between patients with and without neuropathy. However, because these techniques cannot localize peripheral nerve lesions, they are not useful for diagnosing specific entrapment neuropathies.[33]

Other Diagnostic Tests

Some studies have suggested that magnetic resonance neurography[34] and ultrasonography[35] may have utility in the diagnosis of CTS. However, these tests have not been shown to be more accurate than EDS in high-quality studies.[36,37] The department does not cover these services.

TREATMENT OF CARPAL TUNNEL SYNDROME
Conservative Treatment

A critical element for any conservative CTS intervention is to document improved function and ability to return to work (RTW). Because findings of median nerve involvement on NCV strongly predict a good outcome with CTS surgery, any worker suspected of median nerve involvement or with documented increased median nerve latencies who does not gain meaningful and sustainable functional improvement within 6 to 8 weeks of any conservative intervention or combination of interventions should be referred to a specialist or surgeon. To date, although most studies have demonstrated meaningful and significant short-term benefit, better-designed longer-term follow-up studies are needed to clarify the sustainability of relief. Surgical decompression is more effective in general than conservative measures but with potentially more complications and side effects.[38]

Several conservative interventions have demonstrated utility in reducing symptoms and improving function in the short term:

1. Neutral position wrist splits used nocturnally and intermittently during work exposures have been shown to be effective in reducing symptoms, in increasing grip strength, and in improving NCV.[39–42] Studies report that 30% to 70% of patients respond favorably within several months of initiating this intervention. There is no clear evidence on the effectiveness of one splint design over another.[42]
2. Glucocorticoids: Local steroid injections into the carpal tunnel have been demonstrated to provide good short-term relief of CTS.[43,44] About half of all patients receiving this treatment require surgery within 1 year. No more than 2 injections should be given. Oral steroids are not recommended. Although there can be a short-term benefit from oral steroids, the risk of serious adverse effects (eg, avascular necrosis) likely outweighs the benefits.
3. Exercise and mobilization interventions, such as forearm/wrist stretching home exercise regimens, may be of benefit, but the evidence basis for this type of treatment is weak.[45]

Occupational-centered interventions to reduce exposure are believed to be of value, based primarily on epidemiologic studies and consensus opinion.[46,47]

Job modification: Reducing the intensity of manual tasks when feasible may prevent progression and promote recovery from CTS. In most cases, the patient can continue working during conservative treatment. If job modification is not possible or if the patient cannot continue working despite conservative treatment, then surgical CTR should be considered as a treatment option.

The following treatments are not recommended for CTS because there is inadequate or conflicting evidence concerning their effectiveness[41,46]:

1. Vitamin B$_6$ (pyridoxine)
2. Oral diuretics
3. Magnets (not covered per WAC 296-20-03002)
4. Lasers (not covered)
5. Botulinum toxin injections (not covered per WAC 296-20-03002; not approved by the US Food and Drug and Administration for CTS)
6. Iontophoresis (Not covered per WAC 296-20-03002)

Surgical Carpal Tunnel Release

For patients with CTS confirmed by electrodiagnostic studies (EDS), carpal tunnel surgery is more effective in relieving symptoms than conservative treatment such as splinting.[38,39] Decompression of the median nerve at the wrist with release of the transverse carpal ligament is the surgical procedure of choice and can be effectively performed by either open or endoscopic approaches.[47–50] Both are covered by the department. There is no quality evidence that tenosynovectomy, internal neurolysis, and several other adjunct procedures improve the clinical outcome of CTR, and these procedures increase the risk of additional neurologic trauma to the median nerve.[51–54]

All of the following criteria must be met for surgery to be authorized:

1. The clinical presentation is consistent with CTS
2. The EDS criteria for CTS have been met
3. The patient has failed to respond to conservative treatment that included wrist splinting and/or injection

If symptoms return after surgery

Recurring CTS is uncommon. The results of revision surgery are unpredictable. In order to determine whether or not a patient who has had prior CTS surgery is appropriate for revision surgery, at least one of the following criteria should be met:

1. The symptoms and signs should be at least as severe as the preoperative symptoms
2. The result of EDS should be at least as severe as that of preoperative EDS
3. There are electrodiagnostic signs of median nerve worsening

In general, it is helpful to wait at least 6 months from the time of initial surgery before considering revision surgery, unless there are signs of significant surgical complication. This waiting period allows adequate time for healing, scar maturation, rehabilitation, and clinical improvement.

RETURN TO WORK
Early Assessment

In the United States, approximately 7% of workers with upper extremity musculoskeletal disorders account for 75% of the disability in this population.[55] A large prospective study of work-related CTS in the WA workers' compensation system identified several important predictors of long-term disability: low expectations of RTW, no offer of a job accommodation, and high physical demands on the job.[56]

Identifying and attending to these risk factors when patients have not returned to work within 2 to 3 weeks of the initial clinical presentation may improve their chances of returning to work.

Timeliness of the CTS diagnosis can be a critical factor influencing RTW. WA workers diagnosed accurately and early were far more likely to RTW than workers whose CTS was diagnosed weeks or months later.[3] Early coordination of care with improved timeliness and effective communication with the workplace is also likely to help prevent long-term disability in CTS. A recent quality improvement project in WA has demonstrated that organized delivery of occupational best practices similar to those listed in **Table 3** can substantially prevent long-term disability when delivered early on after claim initiation.[57] In addition, removing workers from work and placing them on lost time benefits is dramatically associated with increased risk of developing long-term disability.[58]

Returning to Work After Surgery

RTW after surgery should be possible for many patients regardless of whether open or endoscopic release was performed. Average times for returning to work (panel consensus) are within 2 to 4 weeks for clerical and light duty workers and within 5 to 6 weeks for heavy labor workers. These time frames tend to be shorter for endoscopic surgery; time from surgery to RTW or to activities of daily living is approximately 6 days less with endoscopic than with open surgery.[59]

Table 3 Occupational health CTS quality indicators	
Clinical Care Action	**Time Frame**[a]
Early screening for presence/absence of CTS	First health care visit
Documented history of physical work and nonwork exposures and determination of work relatedness	First or second health care visit
Communication with employer regarding return to work via Activity Prescription Form (or provider's Return to Work Form) or phone call	Each visit
Referral to specialist if no RTW or clinical improvement	If >2 wk of time loss occurs or no improvement of symptoms within 6 wk
Specialist visit	Within 1–3 wk of referral
Nerve conduction studies	If the diagnosis of CTS is being considered, schedule studies as soon as possible. If time loss will extend beyond 2 wk, or if surgery is being considered, these tests are required
Referral for assessment of RTW impediments	If time loss of 4–6 wk
Surgical decompression	Within 4–6 wk of determination of need for surgery
Ergonomic assessment of work site	Within 2 wk of first health care visit to (1) assist with work modification and (2) determine if physical hazards may put other workers at risk for CTS

[a] The timing column is anchored in time from claim filing or first provider visit related to CTS complaints.

In several well-designed studies, most patients recovered function and did not have a permanent impairment that would result in disability.[48,50,60] The panel's experience is that many patients can successfully return to the job of injury.

HAND DIAGRAM

A hand diagram of patient reported numbness or other sensory symptoms can help document the specificity of median nerve distribution (**Fig. 1**).

ELECTRODIAGNOSTIC WORKSHEET

Purpose and instructions

1. The purpose of this worksheet (**Fig. 2**) is to help the department's medical and nursing staff interpret electrodiagnostic studies (EDS) that you do for DLI-WA (Washington Department of Labor and Industries) patients. The worksheet should be used only when the main purpose of your study is to evaluate a patient for CTS.

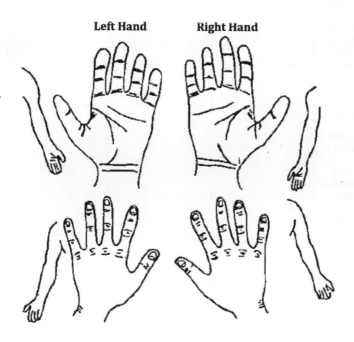

Left Hand   **Right Hand**

This diagram can be printed and completed
by the patient.

Pain	
Tingling	
Numbness	
Decreased Sensation	

Patient Name: _____ Claim#:_____ Date:_____

Comments:

Fig. 1. Hand diagram. (*Courtesy of* Dr Jeffrey N. Katz, Harvard Medical School.)

Technique	Abnormal Values (ms)	Right Arm Value (ms)	Left Arm Value (ms)
1. Median motor distal latency (8 cm) Note: if median motor distal latency is abnormal, then ulnar motor distal latency at 8 cm must be within normal limits(≤3.9 ms)	>4.5		
2. Median sensory distal latency 8 cm recorded (palm to wrist) *or* 14 cm recorded (index, long, or ring finger to wrist) if either of these tests is used alone, at least one other sensory nerve in the ipsilateral hand should be normal	>2.3 >3.6		
3. Median – ulnar motor latency difference (APB vs ADM) at 8 cm	>1.6		
4. Median – ulnar sensory latency difference to digits (14 cm), index or long finger compared to ulnar recorded at the small finger, or median – ulnar difference recorded at the ring finger	>0.5		
5. Median – ulnar sensory latency difference across palm (8 cm)	>0.3		
6. Median – radial sensory latency difference to thumb (10 cm)	>0.6		
7. CSI	>0.9		

Claim number:

Claimant name:

Additional comments:

Signed:
Date:

Fig. 2. Worksheet for carpal tunnel nerve conduction studies.

It is for this reason that the worksheet focuses on distal latency from NCV. It should accompany but not replace the detailed report normally submitted to the department.

2. We encourage you to use the electrodiagnostic worksheet that is appended to this guideline to report EDS results, but the department will accept the results on a report generated by your office system.

3. On the worksheet, sensory distal latency should be measured to response peak and motor distal latency should be measured to response onset.

4. It is not necessary to do all the NCV tests listed on the worksheet. You should do only the studies needed to rule CTS in or out.

5. It is sometimes necessary to do EDS other than the ones listed on the worksheet. If you do any additional studies bearing on the diagnosis of CTS, please write them in the blank area below the listed studies.

6. The value of other studies of median nerve function has not been proven. Those tests are not recommended for the diagnosis of CTS. The following quotation is taken from a literature review published in Muscle & Nerve, 1993, Vol. 16, p. 1392–1414:

Several other variations on median sensory and motor NCV have been reported to be useful for the evaluation of patients with OCTS [occupational carpal tunnel syndrome]. The committee's review of the literature indicated that the value of these tests for the clinical electrodiagnostic evaluation of patients with OCTS remains to be established. These electrodiagnostic studies include the following: (1) studies of the median motor distal latency recorded from the lumbrical muscles, ... (2) measurement of the refractory period of the median nerve, ... (3) median motor residual latency measurements, ... (4) terminal latency ratio, ... (5) median F-wave abnormalities, ... (6) median motor nerve conduction amplitude comparisons with stimulation above and below the carpal ligament, ... (7) anterior interosseous/median nerve latency ratio, ... (8) change in median motor response configuration with median nerve stimulation at the wrist and elbow in the presence of Martin-Gruber anastomosis, ... (9) sensory amplitude measurements, ... and (10) measurement of median sensory and motor nerve conduction across the wrist before and after prolonged wrist flexion.

ACKNOWLEDGMENTS

This guideline was developed in 2008 by Labor and Industries' Industrial Insurance Medical Advisory Committee (IIMAC) and its subcommittee on Upper Extremity Entrapment Neuropathies. Acknowledgment and gratitude go to all subcommittee members, clinical experts, and consultants who contributed to this important guideline:

IIMAC Committee Members: Gregory T. Carter, MD, MS; Dianna Chamblin, MD—Chair; G.A. DeAndrea, MD, MBA; J Ordan Firestone, MD, PhD, MPH; Andrew Friedman, MD.

Subcommittee Clinical Experts: Christopher H. Allan, MD; Douglas P. Hanel, MD; Michel Kliot, MD; Lawrence R. Robinson, MD; Thomas E. Trumble, MD; Nicholas B. Vedder, MD; Michael D. Weiss, MD.

Consultation Provided by: Terrell Kjerulf, MD, Qualis Health; Ken O'Bara, MD, Qualis Health; Scott Carlson, MD; Jeffrey (Jerry) G. Jarvik, MD.

Department staff who helped develop and prepare this guideline include: Gary M. Franklin, MD, MPH, Medical Director; Simone P. Javaher, BSN, MPA, Occupational Nurse Consultant; Reshma N. Kearney, MPH, Epidemiologist; Bintu Marong BS, MS, Epidemiologist.

REFERENCES

1. Latinovic R, Gulliford MC, Hughes RA. Incidence of common compressive neuropathies in primary care. J Neurol Neurosurg Psychiatry 2006;77:263–5.
2. Blanc PD, Faucett I, Kennedy JJ, et al. Self-reported carpal tunnel syndrome: predictors of work disability from the National Health Interview Survey Occupational Health Supplement. Am J Ind Med 1996;30:362–8.
3. Daniell WE, Fulton-Kehoe D, Chiou LA, et al. Work-related carpal tunnel syndrome in Washington State workers' compensation: temporal trends, clinical practices, and disability. Am J Ind Med 2005;48:259–69.
4. Leigh JP, Miller TR. Occupational illnesses within two national data sets. Int J Occup Environ Health 1998;4:99–113.
5. Franklin GM. Peripheral neuropathy. In: Nelson LM, Tanner CM, Van Den Eeden SK, et al, editors. Neuroepidemiology: from principles to practice. New York: Oxford University Press; 2004. p. 279–302.
6. Silverstein B, Welp E, Nelson N, et al. Claims incidence of work-related disorders of the upper extremities. Am J Public Health 1998;88:1827–33.
7. Lawrence RC, Felson DT, Helmick CG, et al. Estimates of the prevalence of arthritis and other rheumatic conditions in the United States. Part II. Arthritis Rheum 2008;58:26–35.
8. Luckhaupt SE, Dalhamer JM, Ward BW, et al. Prevalence and work-relatedness of carpal tunnel syndrome in the working population, United States, 2010 National Health Interview Survey. Am J Ind Med 2013;56:615–24.
9. Jain NB, Higgins LD, Losina E, et al. Epidemiology of musculoskeletal upper extremity ambulatory surgery in the United States. BMC Musculoskelet Disord 2014;15:4.
10. Franklin GM, Haug J, Heyer N, et al. Occupational carpal tunnel syndrome in Washington State, 1984–1988. Am J Ind Med 1991;81:741–6.
11. Stevens J, Beard CM, O'Failon WM, et al. Conditions associated with carpal tunnel syndrome. Mayo Clin Proc 1992;67:541–8.
12. Hakim AJ, Cherkas L, El Zayat S, et al. The genetic contribution to carpal tunnel syndrome in women: a twin study. Arthritis Rheum 2002;47:275–9.
13. Palmer KT, Harris EC, Coggon D. Carpal tunnel syndrome and its relation to occupation: a systematic literature review. Occup Med (Lond) 2007;57:57–66.
14. Shiri R, Miranda H, Heliiovaara M, et al. Physical work load factors and carpal tunnel syndrome: a population-based study. Occup Environ Med 2009;66:368–73.
15. Barcenilla A, March LM, Chen JS, et al. Carpal tunnel syndrome and its relationship to occupation: a meta-analysis. Rheumatology 2012;51:250–61.
16. Andersen JH, Thomsen JF, Overgaard E, et al. Computer use and carpal tunnel syndrome: a 1-year follow-up study. JAMA 2003;289:2963–9.
17. Ali KM, Sathiyasekaran BW. Computer professionals and carpal tunnel syndrome. Int J Occup Saf Ergon 2006;12:319–25.
18. Eleftheriou A, Rachiotis G, Varitimidis S, et al. Cumulative keyboard strokes: a possible risk factor for carpal tunnel syndrome. J Occup Med Toxicol 2012;7:16.
19. Stevens JC, Witt JC, Smith BE, et al. The frequency of carpal tunnel syndrome in computer users at a medical facility. Neurology 2001;56:1568–70.
20. Thomsen JF, Gerr F, Atroshi I. Carpal tunnel syndrome and the use of computer mouse and keyboard: a systematic review. BMC Musculoskelet Disord 2008;9:134.
21. Mediouni Z, de Roquemaurel A, Dumontier C, et al. Is carpal tunnel syndrome related to computer exposure at work? A review and meta-analysis. J Occup Environ Med 2014;56(2):204–8.

22. Rempel D, Evanoff B, Amadio PC, et al. Consensus criteria for the classification of carpal tunnel syndrome in epidemiologic studies. Am J Public Health 1998; 88(10):1447–51.
23. Katz JN, Stirrat CR. A self-administered hand diagram for the diagnosis of carpal tunnel syndrome. J Hand Surg 1990;15A:360–3.
24. Higgs PE, Edwards DF, Martin DS, et al. Relation of preoperative nerve-conduction values to outcome in workers with surgically treated carpal tunnel syndrome. J Hand Surg Am 1997;22:216–21.
25. Coggon D, Ntani G, Harris EC, et al. Impact of carpal tunnel surgery according to pre-operative abnormality of sensory conduction in median nerve: a longitudinal study. BMC Musculoskelet Disord 2013;14:241.
26. Prakash KM, Fook-Chong S, Leoh TH, et al. Sensitivities of sensory nerve conduction study parameters in carpal tunnel syndrome. J Clin Neurophysiol 2006; 23(6):565–7.
27. Buschbacher RM. Median nerve motor conduction to the abductor pollicis brevis. Am J Phys Med Rehabil 1999;78(6 Suppl):S1–8.
28. Sander HW, Quinto C, Saadeh PB, et al. Median and ulnar palm-wrist studies. Clin Neurophysiol 1999;110(8):1462–5.
29. Grossar EA, Prahlow ND, Buschbacher RM. Acceptable difference in sensory and motor latencies between the median and ulnar nerves. J Long Term Eff Med Implants 2006;16(5):395–400.
30. Berkson A, Lohman J, Buschbacher RM. Comparison of median and radial sensory studies to the thumb. J Long Term Eff Med Implants 2006;16(5):387–94.
31. Robinson LR, Micklesen PJ, Wang L. Strategies for analyzing nerve conduction data: superiority of a summary index over single tests. Muscle Nerve 1998;21: 1166–71.
32. Robinson LR. Electrodiagnosis of carpal tunnel syndrome. Phys Med Rehabil Clin N Am 2007;18:733–46.
33. Shy ME, Frohman EM, So YT, et al. Quantitative sensory testing: report on the therapeutics and technology assessment subcommittee of the American Academy of Neurology. Neurology 2003;60:898–904.
34. Jarvik JG, Yuen E, Haynor DR, et al. MR nerve imaging in a prospective cohort of patients with suspected carpal tunnel syndrome. Neurology 2002;58: 1597–602.
35. Wong SM, Griffith JF, Hui ACF, et al. Carpal tunnel syndrome: diagnostic usefulness of sonography. Radiology 2004;232:93–9.
36. Descatha A, Huard L, Aubert F, et al. Meta-analysis on the performance of sonography for the diagnosis of carpal tunnel syndrome. Semin Arthritis Rheum 2012; 41(6):914–22.
37. Fowler JR, Gaughan JP, Ilyas AM. The sensitivity and specificity of ultrasound for the diagnosis of carpal tunnel syndrome: a meta-analysis. Clin Orthop Relat Res 2011;469(4):1089–94.
38. Shi Q, MacDermid JC. Is surgical intervention more effective than non-surgical intervention for carpal tunnel syndrome? A systematic review. J Orthop Surg Res 2011;6:17.
39. Gerritsen AA, de Vet HC, Scholten RJ, et al. Splinting vs surgery in the treatment of carpal tunnel syndrome: a randomized controlled trial. JAMA 2002;288(10): 1245–51.
40. Nobuta S, Sato K, Nakagawa T, et al. Effects of wrist splinting for carpal tunnel syndrome and motor nerve conduction measurements. Ups J Med Sci 2008; 113(2):181–92.

41. O'Connor D, Marshall S, Massy-Westropp N. Non-surgical treatment (other than steroid injection) for carpal tunnel syndrome. Cochrane Database Syst Rev 2003;(1):CD003219.

42. Page MJ, Massy-Westropp N, O'Connor D, et al. Splinting for carpal tunnel syndrome. Cochrane Database Syst Rev 2012;(7):CD010003.

43. American Academy of Orthopedic Surgeons (AAOS). Carpal tunnel syndrome guideline. 2007. Available at: http://www.aaos.org/research/guidelines/guide. asp. Accessed September 24, 2008.

44. Marshall S, Tardif G, Ashworth N. Local corticosteroid injection for carpal tunnel syndrome. Cochrane Database Syst Rev 2012;(1):CD009601.

45. Page MJ, O'Connor D, Pitt V, Massy-Westropp N. Exercise and mobilization interventions for carpal tunnel syndrome. Cochrane Database Syst Rev 2012;(6):CD009899.

46. Verhagen AP, Karels C, Bierma-Zeinstra SM, et al. Ergonomic and physiotherapeutic interventions for treating work-related complaints of the arm, neck or shoulder in adults. A Cochrane systematic review. Eura Medicophys 2007; 43(3):391–405.

47. De Kesel R, Donceel P, De Smet L. Factors influencing return to work after surgical treatment for carpal tunnel syndrome. Occup Med (Lond) 2008;58(3):187–90.

48. Trumble TE, Diao E, Abrams RA, et al. Single-portal endoscopic carpal tunnel release compared with open release: a prospective, randomized trial. J Bone Joint Surg Am 2002;84:1107–15.

49. Palmer DH, Paulson JC, Lane-Larsen CL, et al. Endoscopic carpal tunnel release: a comparison of two techniques with open release. Arthroscopy 1993;9(5): 498–508.

50. Brown RA, Gelberman RH, Seiler JG, et al. Carpal tunnel release: a prospective, randomized assessment of open and endoscopic methods. J Bone Joint Surg Am 1993;9:1265–75.

51. Gelberman RH, Pfeffer GB, Galbraith RT, et al. Results of treatment of severe carpal-tunnel syndrome without internal neurolysis of the median nerve. J Bone Joint Surg Am 1987;69(6):896–903.

52. Mackinnon SE, Dellon AL. Anatomic investigations of nerves at the wrist: I. Orientation of the motor fascicle of the median nerve in the carpal tunnel. Ann Plast Surg 1988;21(1):32–5.

53. Mackinnon SE. Secondary carpal tunnel surgery. Nerurosurg Clin N Am 1991;2: 75–91.

54. Kerr CD, Sybert DR, Albarracin NS. An analysis of the flexor synovium in idiopathic carpal tunnel syndrome: report of 625 cases. J Hand Surg 1992;17(6): 1028–30.

55. Hashemi L, Webster BS, Clance EA, et al. Length of disability and cost of work-related musculoskeletal disorders of the upper extremity. J Occup Environ Med 1998;40:261–9.

56. Turner JA, Franklin G, Fulton-Kehoe D. Early predictors of chronic work disability associated with carpal tunnel syndrome: a longitudinal workers' compensation cohort study. Am J Ind Med 2007;50:489–500.

57. Wickizer T, Franklin G, Fulton-Kehoe D, et al. Improving quality, preventing disability and reducing costs in workers' compensation healthcare: a population-based intervention study. Med Care 2011;49:1105–11.

58. Spector JT, Turner JA, Fulton-Kehoe D, et al. Pre-surgery disability compensation predicts long-term disability among workers with carpal tunnel syndrome. Am J Ind Med 2012;55:816–32.

59. Scholten RJPM, Mink van der Molen A, Uitdehaag BMJ, et al. Surgical treatment options for carpal tunnel syndrome. Cochrane Database Syst Rev 2007;(4):CD003905.
60. Agee JM, McCarroll HR, Tortosa RD, et al. Endoscopic release of the carpal tunnel: a randomized prospective multicenter study. J Hand Surg Am 1992;17: 987–95.

Diagnosis and Treatment of Work-Related Proximal Median and Radial Nerve Entrapment

Gregory T. Carter, MD, MS[a],*, Michael D. Weiss, MD[b]

KEYWORDS

- Proximal median nerve entrapment • Pronator teres syndrome
- Radial nerve entrapment • Posterior interosseous nerve syndrome

KEY POINTS

- Proximal median and radial nerve entrapment are rare conditions.
- A small number of providers make a disproportionate number of these diagnoses, and conduct multiple surgical interventions.
- An accurate diagnosis, including specific electrodiagnostic findings, must be determined.
- Conservative care includes rest, modified activities, splinting at wrist and elbow, physical therapy, antiinflammatory drug therapy, and corticosteroid injections.

INTRODUCTION

Proximal median (PMNE) and radial (RNE) nerve entrapment syndromes are not common. As such, there are no high-quality clinical or scientific studies regarding these conditions. However, these guidelines have been developed using the best available evidence-based studies with an emphasis is on accurate diagnosis and treatment that is curative or rehabilitative. These guidelines were developed originally by the Washington State Labor and Industries' Industrial Insurance Medical Advisory Committee (IIMAC) and its subcommittee on Upper Extremity Entrapment Neuropathies. It focuses on work-related medical conditions. One of the subcommittee's goals is to provide standards that ensure a uniformly high quality of care for injured workers in Washington State. The IIMAC unanimously approved these guidelines, which have been updated recently. The subcommittee that has approved of these guidelines is composed of a group of physicians of various medical specialties, including

a St Luke's Rehabilitation Institute, 711 South Cowley Avenue, Spokane, WA 99202, USA;
b Neuromuscular Division, Department of Neurology, University of Washington School of Medicine, Seattle, 1959 NE, Pacific Avenue, WA 98195, USA
* Corresponding author.
E-mail addresses: gtcarter@uw.edu; CarterG@st-lukes.org

Phys Med Rehabil Clin N Am 26 (2015) 539–549
http://dx.doi.org/10.1016/j.pmr.2015.04.001
1047-9651/15/$ – see front matter © 2015 Elsevier Inc. All rights reserved.

pmr.theclinics.com

rehabilitation medicine, occupational medicine, orthopedic surgery, plastic surgery, neurosurgery, neurology, pain medicine, and electrodiagnostic medicine. The subcommittee based its recommendations on the weight of the best available clinical and scientific evidence from a systematic review of the literature.

Objective confirmation of the diagnosis of PMNE/RNE is critical to making the correct diagnosis and directing appropriate treatment. Entrapment of the median nerve in the proximal forearm must be distinguished from more distal sites of entrapment, such as at the wrist (carpal tunnel) or at the anterior interosseous nerve branch (which supplies no cutaneous sensation). Proximal compression of the median nerve may occur near the antecubital fossa can occur as the nerve traverses any of the following anatomic structures: the ligament of Struthers/supracondylar process, the lacertus fibrosis (bicipital aponeurosis), the fascia of the pronator teres, or the fibrous arch formed by fascia of the flexor digitorum superficialis.[1,2] The anatomy of PMNE is illustrated in **Fig. 1**.

When it occurs in relation to work, RNE usually refers to 1 of 2 syndromes: radial tunnel syndrome or posterior interosseous nerve syndrome (PINS).[3,4] Although RNE may occur from compression at any point along the course of the radial nerve owing to acute trauma (eg, humerus fracture, Saturday night palsy), space-occupying lesion (eg, lipoma, ganglion), or local edema or inflammation, this guideline focuses on radial tunnel syndrome and PINS, which are more typical for RNE arising from repetitive work activities. Radial tunnel syndrome and PINS have been described to occur at 1 of 5 potential sites. These sites, from proximal to distal, include the fibrous bands of the radiocapitellar joint, radial recurrent vessels (the leash of Henry), the tendinous edge of the extensor carpi radialis brevis, the arcade of Frohse, and the distal edge of the supinator. Most cases of RNE have been described at the arcade of Frohse.[3,4] The anatomy of RNE is illustrated in **Fig. 2**.

In general, both work relatedness and appropriate symptoms and signs must be present to accept PMNE on a claim. Electrodiagnostic (EDx) studies, including nerve conduction velocity studies (NCVs) and needle electromyography (EMG), should be scheduled immediately to corroborate the clinical diagnosis. Completion of EDx studies should always be accomplished before any surgery is considered.

CASE DEFINITION

For the purposes of this article, the case definition of confirmed PMNE/RNE included appropriate symptoms, objective physical findings (signs), and abnormal EDx studies. A provisional diagnosis may be made based on appropriate symptoms and objective signs alone, but confirmation of the diagnosis requires abnormal EDx studies. Nonoperative therapy may be considered for cases in which a provisional diagnosis has been made. Operative treatment should be undertaken only in cases where the diagnosis has been confirmed by abnormal EDx studies, because the potential benefits of surgery outweigh the risks.

CLINICAL FINDINGS
Proximal Median Nerve Entrapment

The primary symptom associated with PMNE is pain in the proximal volar area of the forearm. Many patients report an increase in pain severity with an increase in activity. Other symptoms may include weakness in the forearm and the hand (such as a decrease in grip strength), cramping in the hand (writer's cramp), and paresthesia or numbness in the first 3 digits.[5–14] Nocturnal symptoms are not as common for PMNE as they are for carpal tunnel syndrome. There is accompanying tenderness

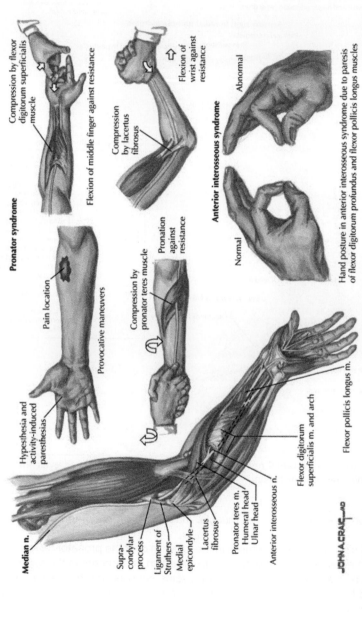

Pronator syndrome

Median n.

Hypesthesia and activity-induced paresthesias

Pain location

Provocative maneuvers

Compression by flexor digitorum superficialis muscle

Flexion of middle finger against resistance

Compression by lacertus fibrosus

Flexion of wrist against resistance

Compression by pronator teres muscle

Pronation against resistance

Anterior interosseous syndrome

Normal

Abnormal

Hand posture in anterior interosseous syndrome due to paresis of flexor digitorum profundus and flexor pollicis longus muscles

Supracondylar process

Ligament of Struthers

Medial epicondyle

Lacertus fibrosus

Pronator teres m.
Humeral head
Ulnar head

Anterior interosseous n.

Flexor digitorum superficialis m. and arch

Flexor pollicis longus m.

JOHN A CRAIG MD

Fig. 1. The anatomy of proximal median nerve entrapment.

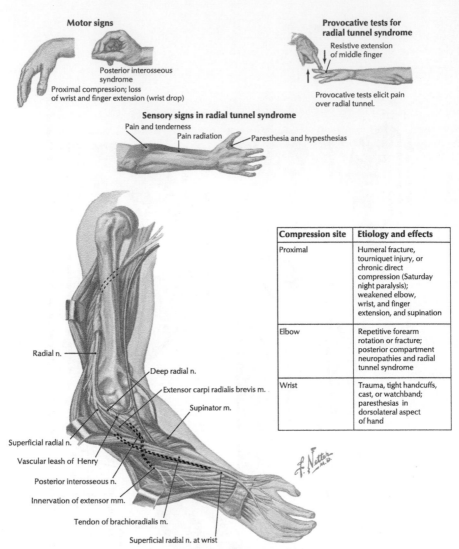

Motor signs

Posterior interosseous syndrome

Proximal compression; loss of wrist and finger extension (wrist drop)

Provocative tests for radial tunnel syndrome

Resistive extension of middle finger

Provocative tests elicit pain over radial tunnel.

Sensory signs in radial tunnel syndrome

Pain and tenderness

Pain radiation

Paresthesia and hypesthesias

Radial n.

Deep radial n.

Extensor carpi radialis brevis m.

Supinator m.

Superficial radial n.

Vascular leash of Henry

Posterior interosseous n.

Innervation of extensor mm.

Tendon of brachioradialis m.

Superficial radial n. at wrist

Compression site	Etiology and effects
Proximal	Humeral fracture, tourniquet injury, or chronic direct compression (Saturday night paralysis); weakened elbow, wrist, and finger extension, and supination
Elbow	Repetitive forearm rotation or fracture; posterior compartment neuropathies and radial tunnel syndrome
Wrist	Trauma, tight handcuffs, cast, or watchband; paresthesias in dorsolateral aspect of hand

Fig. 2. The anatomy of radial nerve entrapment. Copyright © 2015 Elsevier Inc. All rights reserved. www.netterimages.com.

to palpation over pronator teres muscle. Inability to produce an "OK" sign may be noted.

Physical signs include tenderness in the forearm over the pronator teres muscle and along the median nerve distribution. Unlike median entrapment at the carpal tunnel, if weakness is present, it should involve muscles supplied by the median nerve both above and below the wrist. The Tinel sign (paresthesias radiating in a median nerve distribution with pressure or tapping over the median nerve in the forearm) may be present, but by itself is not specifically diagnostic of PMNE. A positive Phalen sign (paresthesias radiating in a median nerve distribution with sustained flexion of the wrist) or Tinel sign with tapping over the wrist more likely indicates carpal tunnel syndrome, rather than PMNE.

Three provocative tests have been described to help corroborate the site of compression for PMNE.[15] These provocative tests do not replace the objective signs discussed elsewhere in this article. The sensitivity and specificity of these provocative tests have not been established. The tests are based on creating maximal tension on the anatomic sites that can contribute to PMNE:

1. The pronator teres muscle is implicated if symptoms are reproduced upon resisted pronation of the forearm in neutral position with the elbow extended.
2. The lacertus fibrosis (bicipital aponeurosis) is implicated if symptoms are reproduced upon resisted elbow flexion at 120° to 130° flexion with the forearm in maximal supination.
3. The flexor digitorum superficialis is implicated if symptoms are reproduced upon resisted flexion of the proximal interphalangeal joint to the long finger ("middle finger flexion test").[13–15]

Symptoms associated with RNE may include weakness in radial innervated muscles and pain or aching over the proximal, lateral forearm. Patients may report an increase in pain severity with an increase with activity or during sleep. Loss of motor function is most common with PINS.[16]

Signs on examination may include tenderness over the radial nerve distal to the lateral epicondyle. Tenderness on palpation is a useful objective finding, but alone cannot support the diagnosis of RNE. Motor findings include difficulty extending the thumb, fingers, or wrist.[17] Motor testing should compare strength of radial innervated muscles to strength of the same muscles in the nonaffected limb as well as nonradial innervated muscles of the affected limb. Atrophy of affected muscles may be seen in chronic or severe cases.

Provocative tests have been described to help corroborate the diagnosis of RNE. These tests include pressure over the radial tunnel ("radial nerve compression test"), resisted supination with the elbow extended ("resisted supination test"), and resisted extension of the middle finger at the metacarpophalangeal joint ("middle finger test"). These tests are based on creating maximal tension on the anatomic sites that are involved in RNE.[18] However, the sensitivity and specificity of these tests have not been established. Every effort should be made to confirm objectively the diagnosis of RNE before considering surgery. A differential diagnosis for RNE includes extensor tendinitis and lateral epicondylitis (which can coexist with RNE), neuralgic amyotrophy, brachial plexopathy, or cervical radiculopathy.[18,19]

ESTABLISHING WORK RELATEDNESS

Work-related activities may cause or contribute to the development of PMNE/RNE. Establishing work relatedness requires all of the following:

1. Exposure: Workplace activities that contribute to or cause PMNE/RNE, and
2. Outcome: A diagnosis of PMNE/RNE that meets the diagnostic criteria, and
3. Relationship: Generally accepted scientific evidence, which establishes on a more probable than not basis (>50%) that the workplace activities (exposure) in an individual case contributed to the development or worsening of the condition (outcome).

Work-related PMNE is associated most often with activities requiring extensive, repetitive, forceful, or prolonged use of the elbow or forearm. Examples of this include heavy labor using vibrating hand tools; repetitive grasping; prolonged hammering; lifting, carrying, and placing heavy objects; and repetitive scraping or packaging motions. Typical occupations that place a worker at risk for PMNE include assembly line worker, cashier, carpenter, cook, mechanic, barber, concrete or wood worker, and dentistry, including dental hygienist.

Certain work-related activities have been associated with RNE, usually those requiring forceful and repetitive elbow extension and forearm supination, handling of loads greater than 1 kg, and firm pinching or squeezing of objects or hand tools.[20,21] Jobs where these activities occur often may include but are not limited to the following: truck driver, cement or brick layer, assembly line worker, automobile brakes industry worker, television industry worker, shoes and clothing industry worker, mechanic, ice cream packer, seamstress, secretary, construction smelting, machine tuning, assembly line inspection, and sewing packing.[20,22–24] This is not intended as an exhaustive list and is meant only as a guide in the consideration of work relatedness.[24–26]

ELECTRODIAGNOSTIC STUDIES

EDx studies are required to objectively confirm the diagnosis of both PMNE and RNE. This includes NCVs and needle EMG. These studies are useful both to diagnose PMNE/RNE and also to rule out other forms of nerve compression or injury. For example, unlike the distal median nerve entrapment within the carpal tunnel, NCVs in PMNE are often normal.[11,12] Short segment nerve conduction studies have not been demonstrated to diagnose this entity reliably. However, EMG studies may show an abnormality in the distribution of the proximal median nerve of the forearm. The diagnosis is confirmed specifically by EMG demonstrating membrane instability (eg, increased insertional activity, fibrillation potentials, positive sharp waves) of median innervated muscles both below and above the wrist in the forearm (unlike carpal tunnel syndrome, which should only affect median innervated muscles below the wrist).[11] The median and radial nerve innervated muscles are listed in **Boxes 1** and **2**.

Box 1
Median nerve innervated muscles

Forearm: main branch

- Pronator teres

- Flexor carpi radialis

- Flexor digitorum profundus (medial half)

- Flexor digitorum superficialis

- Palmaris longus

Forearm: anterior interosseous nerve

- Flexor pollicis longus

- Pronator quadratus

- Flexor digitorum profundus (lateral half)

Hand

- Abductor pollicis brevis

- Flexor pollicis brevis

- Opponens pollicis

- Lumbricals (index and middle)

> **Box 2**
> **Radial nerve innervated muscles**
>
> *Forearm: deep branch*
> - Externsor carpi radialis brevis
> - Supinator
>
> *Forearm: posterior interosseous nerve*
> - Extensor digitorum communis
> - Extensor digiti minimi
> - Extensor carpi ulnaris
> - Abductor pollicis longus
> - Extensor pollicis longus and brevis
> - Extensor indicis proprius
>
> *Arm: muscular branch*
> - Triceps brachii (medial, lateral and long heads)
> - Anconeus
> - Brachioradialis
> - Extensor carpi radialis longus

EMG criteria that confirm the diagnosis of PMNE include evidence of denervation (eg, increased insertional activity, fibrillation potentials, positive sharp waves) as follows: Needle EMG abnormalities noted in a muscle supported by the anterior interosseous nerve (flexor pollicis longus, pronator quadratus, or radial aspect of the flexor digitorum profundus) or a median innervated muscle in the forearm (pronator teres, flexor carpi radialis, flexor digitorum superficialis). In addition, there must be abnormalities noted in a median innervated muscle in the hand (abductor pollicis brevis, flexor pollicis brevis, or opponens pollicis). Moreover, there should be no abnormalities noted in EMG of muscles supplied by the ulnar or radial nerve.

A pure anterior interosseous nerve entrapment would only show EMG abnormalities in the flexor pollicis longus, pronator quadratus, or radial aspect of the flexor digitorum profundus.[11]

For RNE NCVs abnormalities, such as radial motor or sensory conduction block across the elbow, or reduced sensory nerve action potentials, are of unproven utility; therefore, NCV alone should not be relied upon to confirm the diagnosis. EDx confirmation requires abnormal EMG, with evidence of denervation in muscles supplied by the posterior interosseous nerve with or without denervation in other radially innervated forearm muscles. EDx studies should exclude other potential causes of neuropathic symptoms, such as cervical radiculopathy, brachial plexopathy, or neuralgic amyotrophy. RNE may be confused with enthesitis of the epicondyle muscle insertions (an entity often occurring simultaneously), or even treatment-resistant epicondylitis.

Muscles innervated by the muscular branch of radial nerve in the arm include the triceps brachii (long head, medial head, lateral head), anconeous, brachioradialis, and the extensor carpi radialis longus. The deep branch of the radial nerve innervates the following muscles in the forearm: extensor carpi radialis brevis and the supinator. In the forearm, the posterior interosseous branch of the radial nerve innervates these muscles: extensor digitorum communis, extensor digiti minimi, extensor carpi ulnaris, abductor pollicis longus, extensor pollicis brevis, extensor pollicis longus, and the extensor indicis proprius.

OTHER DIAGNOSTIC TESTS

The scientific evidence is insufficient to support the use of MRI/neurography, or ultrasonography in the diagnosis of either PMNE or RNE.[27–30]

TREATMENT
Conservative Treatment

Conservative treatment for both PMNE and RNE has been described only in narrative reviews, case reports, and retrospective case series. Examples include rest, modification of activities that exacerbate symptoms, splinting at wrist and elbow, physical therapy, antiinflammatory drug therapy, and corticosteroid injections.[31–35] Patients do not usually need time off from work activities before surgery unless they present with objective weakness or sensory loss in the distribution of the proximal median nerve that limits work activities or poses a substantial safety risk. Conservative care should be ongoing for at least 6 weeks.

Surgical Treatment

Every effort should be made to verify objectively the diagnosis of PMNE/RNE before considering surgery. One potentially competing diagnosis is neuralgic amyotrophy, which may mimic these syndromes. This condition often produces more widespread abnormalities affecting multiple upper extremity nerves. In addition, it is usually accompanied by proximal pain around the shoulder girdle, rather than in the forearm. This condition usually improves spontaneously in 6 to 12 months. This idiopathic condition would not normally be considered a work-related condition. Without confirmation of nerve compression by both objective clinical findings and abnormal EDx studies, surgery should not be performed.

Surgical treatment for PMNE has been described only in narrative reviews, case reports, and retrospective case series. Surgical treatment should only be considered if the condition does not improve despite conservative treatment, or if the condition interferes with work or activities of daily living. Surgical treatment is only indicated in patients who have appropriate symptoms and 1 or more of the objective clinical findings described elsewhere in this article in addition to abnormal electrodiagnostic studies (EDS). Surgery should include exploration of the median nerve throughout its proximal course and release of all compressive structures, which may include the ligament of Struthers (if it is present), the lacertus fibrosis (bicipital aponeurosis), the fascia of the pronator teres, and the fascia of the flexor digitorum superficialis.[31–34] Although complete release may require nerve decompression at multiple sites, this is considered a single procedure.

In rare cases with long-standing motor palsy of part or all of the median nerve, tendon transfers may be considered to hasten return to function. When a complete palsy has been present for 1 or more muscles for 3 or more months, the patient and the surgeon should consider the options for tendon transfers. In patients who have already had a decompression of the proximal median nerve 6 months or more previously with incomplete return of motor function, repeat EDx studies are recommended. If the EDx studies show no improvement or worse neurologic function, a reexploration may be necessary. Patients with PMNE rarely present with prominent sensory symptoms. For patients with a preoperative loss of sensation who do not have recovery of sensation 6 months or more after surgical treatment, repeat EDx studies are recommended. If these studies show no improvement or worse neurologic function, a reexploration may be necessary.

Surgical treatment for RNE has been described in narrative reviews, case reports, and retrospective case series.[35–41] Surgery should include exploration of the radial nerve throughout its course to decompress it by resecting any compressive and/or constrictive structures. These may include any of the 5 sites of compression mentioned elsewhere in this article. No specific method of surgical treatment has been proven to be most effective.

RETURN TO WORK
Early Assessment

Among workers with upper extremity disorders, 7% of workers account for 75% of the long-term disability.[42] A large prospective study in the Washington State workers' compensation system identified several important predictors of long-term disability: low expectations of return to work (RTW), no offer of a job accommodation, and high physical demands on the job.[43,44] Identifying and attending to these risk factors when patients have not returned to work within 2 to 3 weeks of the initial clinical presentation may improve their chances of RTW.

The timeliness of the diagnosis can be a critical factor influencing RTW. Washington State workers diagnosed accurately and early were far more likely to RTW than workers whose condition was diagnosed weeks or months later. Early coordination of care with improved timeliness and effective communication with the workplace is also likely to help prevent long-term disability. A suggested treatment algorithm with timing of interventions is noted in **Fig. 2.**

Returning to Work After Surgery

Most patients requiring a PMNE release alone can return to light duty work in approximately 3 weeks and regular duty work in approximately 6 weeks. A course of hand therapy may help functional recovery and is particularly important for patients requiring tendon transfers or for patients with residual weakness. These patients may return to light duty work in approximately 6 to 8 weeks and regular duty work in approximately 10 to 12 weeks.

REFERENCES

1. Olehnik WK, Manske PR, Szerzinski J. Median nerve compression in the proximal forearm. J Hand Surg Am 1994;19(1):121–6.
2. Hartz CR, Linscheid RL, Gramse RR, et al. The pronator teres syndrome: compressive neuropathy of the median nerve. J Bone Joint Surg Am 1981; 63(6):885–90.
3. Kim DH, Murovic JA, Kim YY, et al. Surgical treatment and outcomes in 45 cases of posterior interosseous nerve entrapments and injuries. J Neurosurg 2006; 104(5):766–77.
4. Plate AM, Green SM. Compressive radial neuropathies. Instr Course Lect 2000; 49:295–304.
5. Eversmann WW. Proximal median nerve compression. Hand Clin 1992;8(2):307–15.
6. Lee MJ, LaStayo PC. Pronator syndrome and other nerve compressions that mimic carpal tunnel syndrome. J Orthop Sports Phys Ther 2004;34(10):601–9.
7. Lacey SH, Soldatis JJ. Bilateral pronator syndrome associated with anomalous heads of the pronator teres muscle: a case report. J Hand Surg Am 1993; 18(2):349–51.

8. Morris HH, Peters BH. Pronator syndrome: clinical and electrophysiological features in seven cases. J Neurol Neurosurg Psychiatr 1976;39(5):461–4.
9. Stal M, Hagert CG, Englund JE. Pronator syndrome: a retrospective study of median nerve entrapment at the elbow in female machine milkers. J Agric Saf Health 2004;10(4):247–56.
10. Wiggins CE. Pronator syndrome. South Med J 1982;75(2):240–1.
11. Bridgeman C, Naidu S, Kothari MJ. Clinical and electrophysiological presentation of pronator syndrome. Electromyogr Clin Neurophysiol 2007;47(2):89–92.
12. Gross PT, Jones HR Jr. Proximal median neuropathies: electromyographic and clinical correlation. Muscle Nerve 1992;15(3):390–5.
13. Johnson RK, Spinner M, Shrewsbury MM. Median nerve entrapment syndrome in the proximal forearm. J Hand Surg Am 1979;4(1):48–51.
14. Rehak DC. Pronator syndrome. Clin Sports Med 2001;20(3):531–40.
15. Mysiew WJ, Colachis SC. The pronator syndrome. An evaluation of dynamic maneuvers for improving electrodiagnostic sensitivity. Am J Phys Med Rehabil 1991; 70(5):274–7.
16. Bolster MA, Bakker XR. Radial tunnel syndrome: emphasis on the superficial branch of the radial nerve. J Hand Surg Eur Vol 2009;34(3):343–7.
17. Lubahn JD, Cermak MB. Uncommon nerve compression syndromes of the upper extremity. J Am Acad Orthop Surg 1998;6(6):378–86.
18. Sarris IK, Papadimitriou NG, Sotereanos DG. Radial tunnel syndrome. Tech Hand Up Extrem Surg 2002;6(4):209–12.
19. Mondelli M, Morano P, Ballerini M, et al. Mononeuropathies of the radial nerve: clinical and neurographic findings in 91 consecutive cases. J Electromyogr Kinesiol 2005;15:377–83.
20. Roquelaure Y, Raimbeau G, Dano C, et al. Occupational risk factors for radial tunnel syndrome in industrial workers. Scand J Work Environ Health 2000;26(6): 507–13.
21. van Rijn RM, Huisstede BM, Koes BW, et al. Associations between work related factors and specific disorders at the elbow: a systematic literature review. Rheumatology (Oxford) 2009;48(5):528–36.
22. Fardin P, Negrin P, Sparta S, et al. Posterior interosseous nerve neuropathy: clinical and electromyographical aspects. Electromyogr Clin Neurophysiol 1992;32: 229–34.
23. Jebson PJ, Engber WD. Radial tunnel syndrome: long-term results of surgical decompression. J Hand Surg Am 1997;22(5):889–96.
24. Kupfer DM, Bronson J, Lee GW, et al. Differential latency testing: a more sensitive test for radial tunnel syndrome. J Hand Surg Am 1998;23(5):859–64.
25. Lee JT, Azari K, Jones NF. Long term results of radial tunnel release–the effect of co-existing tennis elbow, multiple compression syndromes and workers' compensation. J Plast Reconstr Aesthet Surg 2008;61(9):1095–9.
26. Verhaar J, Spaans F. Radial tunnel syndrome. An investigation of compression neuropathy as a possible cause. J Bone Joint Surg Am 1991;73(4):539–44.
27. Thawait GK, Subhawong TK, Thawait SK, et al. Magnetic resonance neurography of median neuropathies proximal to the carpal tunnel. Skeletal Radiol 2012;41(6): 623–32.
28. Andreisek G, Burg D, Studer A, et al. Upper extremity peripheral neuropathies: role and impact of MR imaging on patient management. Eur Radiol 2008;18(9): 1953–61.
29. Subhawong TK, Wang KC, Thawait SK, et al. High resolution imaging of tunnels by magnetic resonance neurography. Skeletal Radiol 2012;41(1):15–31.

30. Ferdinand BD, Rosenberg ZS, Schweitzer ME, et al. MR imaging features of radial tunnel syndrome: initial experience. Radiology 2006;240(1):161–8.

31. Floranda EE, Jacobs BC. Evaluation and treatment of upper extremity nerve entrapment syndromes. Prim Care 2013;40(4):925–43.

32. Simon Perez C, García Medrano B, Rodriguez Mateos JI, et al. Radial tunnel syndrome: results of surgical decompression by a postero-lateral approach. Int Orthop 2014;38(10):2129–35.

33. Tsai P, Steinberg DR. Median and radial nerve compression about the elbow. Instr Course Lect 2008;57:177–85.

34. Leclère FM, Bignion D, Franz T, et al. Endoscopically assisted nerve decompression of rare nerve compression syndromes at the upper extremity. Arch Orthop Trauma Surg 2013;133(4):575–82.

35. Hagert E, Hagert CG. Upper extremity nerve entrapments: the axillary and radial nerves–clinical diagnosis and surgical treatment. Plast Reconstr Surg 2014; 134(1):71–80.

36. Knutsen EJ, Calfee RP. Uncommon upper extremity compression neuropathies. Hand Clin 2013;29(3):443–53.

37. Huisstede B, Miedema HS, van Opstal T, et al. Interventions for treating the radial tunnel syndrome: a systematic review of observational studies. J Hand Surg Am 2008;33(1):72–8.

38. Atroshi I, Johnsson R, Ornstein E. Radial tunnel release. Unpredictable outcome in 37 consecutive cases with a 1-5 year follow-up. Acta Orthop Scand 1995;66(3): 255–7.

39. Sotereanos DG, Varitimidis SE, Giannakopoulos PN, et al. Results of surgical treatment for radial tunnel syndrome. J Hand Surg Am 1999;24(3):566–70.

40. De Smet L, Van Raebroeckx T, Van Ransbeeck H. Radial tunnel release and tennis elbow: disappointing results? Acta Orthop Belg 1999;65(4):510–3.

41. Rinker B, Effron CR, Beasley RW. Proximal radial compression neuropathy. Ann Plast Surg 2004;52(2):174–80.

42. Hashemi L, Webster BS, Clance EA, et al. Length of disability and cost of work-related musculoskeletal disorders of the upper extremity. J Occup Environ Med 1998;40:261–9.

43. Turner JA, Franklin G, Fulton-Kehoe D. Early predictors of chronic work disability associated with carpal tunnel syndrome: a longitudinal workers' compensation cohort study. Am J Ind Med 2007;50:489–500.

44. Wickizer TM, Franklin G, Fulton-Kehoe D, et al. Improving quality, preventing disability and reducing costs in workers' compensation healthcare: a population-based intervention study. Med Care 2011;49(12):1105–11.

Work-Related Neurogenic Thoracic Outlet Syndrome
Diagnosis and Treatment

Gary M. Franklin, MD, MPH[a,b,c,d],*

KEYWORDS

- Diagnosis • Practice guidelines • Thoracic outlet syndrome • Treatment
- Workers' compensation

KEY POINTS

- The diagnosis and treatment of neurogenic thoracic outlet syndrome (NTOS) are highly controversial and associated with surgical interventions based on no clear-cut evidence of presence of true thoracic outlet syndrome (TOS).
- Considering the poor outcomes reported from the surgical management of NTOS in most workers' compensation cases, this guideline requires objective evidence of brachial plexus disorder, including abnormal electrodiagnostic tests.
- In workers' compensation, a majority of patients have poor outcomes of surgery for NTOS 1 year after surgery.
- Approximately 20% of patients may have new adverse outcomes, primarily related to new neurologic complaints or lung pathology, the most serious of which is phrenic nerve dysfunction.

INTRODUCTION

This guideline is to be used by physicians, claim managers, occupational nurses, and utilization review staff. The emphasis is on accurate diagnosis and treatment that are curative or rehabilitative (see http://app.leg.wa.gov/WAC/default.aspx?cite=296-20-01002 for definitions). An electrodiagnostic worksheet and guideline summary are appended to the end of this document.

This guideline was developed in 2010 by the Washington State Industrial Insurance Medical Advisory Committee (IIMAC) and its subcommittee on Upper Extremity Entrapment Neuropathies. The subcommittee presented its work to the full IIMAC, and the IIMAC voted with full consensus advising the Washington State Department of Labor and Industries to adopt the guideline. This guideline was based on the weight of the best available clinical and scientific evidence from a systematic review of the literature

[a] Washington State Department of Labor and Industries, Olympia, WA 98501, USA; [b] University of Washington, Department of Environmental and Occupational Health Sciences; [c] Department of Neurology; [d] Department of Health Services
* Washington State Department of Labor and Industries, Olympia, WA 98501.
E-mail address: fral235@lni.wa.gov

Phys Med Rehabil Clin N Am 26 (2015) 551–561
http://dx.doi.org/10.1016/j.pmr.2015.04.004
1047-9651/15/$ – see front matter © 2015 Elsevier Inc. All rights reserved.

(evidence was classified using criteria defined by the American Academy of Neurology)[1] and a consensus of expert opinion. One of IIMAC's primary goals is to provide standards that ensure high quality of care for injured workers in Washington State.

TOS is characterized by pain, paresthesias, and weakness in the upper extremity, which may be exacerbated by elevation of the arms or by exaggerated movements of the head and neck. There are 3 categories of thoracic outlet syndrome: arterial, venous, and neurogenic. Arterial and venous thoracic outlet syndromes involve obstruction of the subclavian artery or vein, respectively, as they pass through the thoracic outlet. These vascular categories of TOS should include obvious clinical signs of vascular insufficiency: a cold, pale extremity in cases of arterial TOS, or a swollen, cyanotic extremity in cases of venous TOS. There is a separate surgical guideline for vascular TOS. This guideline focuses solely on nonacute NTOS.

Work-related NTOS occurs due to compression of the brachial plexus, predominantly affecting its lower trunk, at 1 of 3 potential sites. Compression can occur between the anterior scalene muscle (ASM) and middle scalene muscle (or sometimes through the ASM); beneath the clavicle in the costoclavicular space; or beneath the tendon of the pectoralis minor.[2]

The medical literature describes 2 categories of NTOS: true NTOS and disputed NTOS. A diagnosis of true NTOS requires electrodiagnostic study (EDS) abnormalities showing evidence of brachial plexus injury (discussed later). Disputed NTOS describes cases of NTOS for which EDS abnormalities have not been demonstrated. To avoid confusion that has arisen over these categories, this guideline does not use such terms. Rather, it provides guidance regarding treatment of cases of NTOS that have been confirmed by EDS abnormalities compared with those cases for which the provisional diagnosis has not been confirmed by such studies.

In general, work-relatedness and appropriate symptoms and objective signs must be present for the Washington State Department of Labor and Industries to accept NTOS on a claim. EDSs, including nerve conduction velocity studies and needle electromyography (EMG), should be scheduled immediately to confirm the clinical diagnosis. If time loss extends beyond 2 weeks or if surgery is requested, completion of EDSs is required and does not need prior authorization.

ESTABLISHING WORK-RELATEDNESS

Work-related activities may cause or contribute to the development of NTOS.[3,4] Because simply identifying an association with workplace activities is not, in itself, adequate evidence of a causal relationship, establishing work-relatedness requires all of the following:

1. Exposure: workplace activities that contribute to or cause NTOS
2. Outcome: a diagnosis of NTOS that meets the diagnostic criteria (discussed later)
3. Relationship: generally accepted scientific evidence, which establishes on a more probable than not basis (greater than 50%) that the workplace activities (exposure) in an individual case contributed to the development or worsening of the condition (outcome)

When the Washington State Department of Labor and Industries receives notification of an occupational disease, an occupational disease and employment history form is mailed to the worker, employer, or attending provider. The form should be completed and returned to the insurer as soon as possible. If a worker's attending provider completes the form, provides a detailed history in the chart note, and gives an opinion on causality, the provider may be paid for this (use billing code 1055M).

Additional billing information is available in the Attending Doctor's Handbook (Available at: http://www.lni.wa.gov/IPUB/252-004-000.pdf).

Symptoms of NTOS may be exacerbated by certain work-related activities, usually involving elevation or sustained use of the arms. Such activities may include but are not limited to the following[5]:

Lifting overhead
Reaching overhead
Holding tools or objects above shoulder level
Carrying heavy weights

Several occupations have been associated with NTOS. This is not an exhaustive list and is meant only as a guide in the consideration of work-relatedness:

Dry wall hanger or plasterer
Welder
Beautician
Assembly line inspector
Shelf stocker
Dental hygienist

MAKING THE DIAGNOSIS
Symptoms and Signs

A case definition of confirmed NTOS includes appropriate symptoms, objective physical findings (signs), and abnormal EDSs. A provisional diagnosis of NTOS may be made based on appropriate symptoms and objective signs, but confirmation of the diagnosis requires abnormal EDSs.

Classic symptoms of NTOS include pain, paresthesias, and weakness in the upper extremity. Paresthesias most commonly affect the ring and small fingers.[6] Symptom severity tends to increase after certain activities and worsens at the end of the day or during sleep.

Signs on examination may include tenderness to palpation over the brachial plexus, the scalene muscles, the trapezius muscles, or the anterior chest wall. Although tenderness may be a useful objective finding, it cannot support the diagnosis of NTOS alone. Advanced cases of NTOS are characterized by objective signs of weakness of the hand, loss of dexterity of the fingers, and atrophy of the affected muscles.

Provocative tests have been described that may help corroborate the diagnosis of NTOS. These tests are based on creating maximal tension on the anatomic sites of constriction. Studies have found a high false-positive rate for these tests in healthy subjects as well as patients with carpal tunnel syndrome.[7] Although they are described for completeness, the sensitivity and specificity of these tests for NTOS have not been established, and these tests cannot replace confirmatory EDS testing (discussed later).

Provocative tests include

- The elevated arm stress test (or Roos test) — patient places the affected arm in full abduction and external rotation and then opens and closes the hands slowly for 3 minutes. This test constricts the costoclavicular space. It is considered abnormal if typical symptoms are elicited and the patient cannot sustain this activity for the full 3 minutes.
- The Adson test — patient extends the neck and rotates the head toward the involved extremity, which is held extended at the side. This test constricts the interscalene triangle. It is considered abnormal if a change in the radial pulse is detected when the patients inhale deeply and hold their breath.

- The Wright test—patient sits or stands with the arm in full abduction and external rotation. This test constricts the costoclavicular space. It is considered abnormal if typical symptoms are elicited and a change in pulse is detected.
- The costoclavicular test—examiner depresses patient's shoulder. This test constricts the costoclavicular space and creates tension across the pectoralis minor. It is considered abnormal if typical symptoms are elicited.

Every effort should be made to objectively confirm the diagnosis of NTOS before considering surgery. A differential diagnosis for NTOS includes musculoskeletal disease (eg, arthritis or tendinitis) of the cervical spine, shoulder girdle, or arm; cervical radiculopathy or upper extremity nerve entrapment[8]; idiopathic inflammation of the brachial plexus (also known as Parsonage-Turner syndrome); and brachial plexus compression due to an infiltrative process or space-occupying mass (eg, Pancoast tumor of the lung apex).

Electrodiagnostic Studies

EDS abnormalities are required to objectively confirm the diagnosis of NTOS. Given the uncertainties in diagnostic assessment of NTOS, EDSs should be obtained as soon as the diagnosis is considered. EDSs may help gauge the severity of injury.[9–11] EDSs can help exclude conditions that may mimic NTOS, such as ulnar nerve entrapment or cervical radiculopathy.[12] EDS evidence that confirms a diagnosis of NTOS requires

1. Absent or reduced amplitude (<12 uV) of the ulnar antidromic sensory nerve action potential (SNAP) or absent or reduced amplitude (<10 uV) of the medial antebrachial cutaneous nerve (MABC) antidromic SNAP, with normal amplitude of the MABC SNAP in the contralateral (unaffected) extremity and
2. Absent or reduced amplitude (<5 mV) of the median nerve compound motor action potential (CMAP) or absent or prolonged minimum latency (>33 ms) of the ulnar F wave (with or without abnormalities of the median F wave) and with normal F waves in the contralateral (unaffected) upper extremity or needle EMG showing denervation (eg, fibrillation potentials, positive sharp waves) in at least 1 muscle supplied by each of 2 different nerves from the lower trunk of the brachial plexus, with normal EMG of the cervical paraspinal muscles and at least 1 muscle supplied by a nerve from the middle or upper trunk of the brachial plexus. And, to exclude the presence of other focal neuropathies or polyneuropathy as a cause for the abnormalities (described previously), the following must also be shown:
3. Normal amplitude (≥15 uV) of the median nerve antidromic SNAP and
4. Normal conduction velocity (≥50 m/s) of the ulnar motor nerve across the elbow

Other Diagnostic Tests

Arterial or venous vascular studies may be helpful in the diagnosis of suspected arterial or venous TOS. These tests have poor specificity, however, for NTOS, and there is no substantial evidence that vascular studies can reliably confirm the diagnosis of NTOS. Therefore, vascular studies conducted as a diagnostic tool for NTOS are not authorized.

Some investigators have suggested that MRI neurography may be helpful in the diagnosis of NTOS. This service is not authorized for this condition, however, because the clinical utility of these tests has not yet been proved. Although the IIMAC recognizes that this tests may be useful in unusual circumstances where EDS results are normal but there are appropriate clinical symptoms, the IIMAC believes that at this time the use of these tests is investigational and should be used only in a research setting.

ASM blocks have been used in the evaluation of suspected NTOS.[13,14] This test has poor specificity for NTOS, however, and there is no substantial evidence that ASM can reliably confirm the diagnosis of NTOS. Therefore, ASM blocks conducted as a diagnostic tool for NTOS are not authorized.

Radiographs of the chest may be useful to evaluate the possibility of an infiltrative process or space-occupying mass (eg, Pancoast tumor of the lung apex) compressing the brachial plexus.

TREATMENT

Nonsurgical therapy may be considered for cases in which a provisional diagnosis of NTOS has been made. Surgical treatment should be provided only for cases in which a diagnosis of NTOS has been confirmed by abnormal EDSs. Under these circumstances, the potential benefits of brachial plexus decompression may outweigh the risks of surgery.

Conservative Treatment

Conservative treatment of NTOS has been described in narrative reviews, case reports, and retrospective case series.[15–17] No randomized controlled trials have been conducted to measure the efficacy of conservative treatments for NTOS. No specific method of conservative treatment has proved most effective due to a lack of comparative studies.[15] An observational study (n = 50), however, showed that strengthening and stretching exercises reduced pain among 80% of patients after 3 months and among 94% of patients after 6 months,[16] and a 2007 systematic review of the available literature concluded that conservative treatment seems effective in reducing symptoms, improving function, and facilitating return to work (RTW).[15] Examples of conservative treatment include modification of activities that exacerbate symptoms, education, postural exercises, physical therapy, and antiinflammatory drug therapy.

Because surgical outcomes are poor in many situations, conservative interventions, such as stretching and strengthening exercises, should be considered first. If the initial response to conservative treatment is incomplete, modifying or changing the approach should be considered. If there is no response to conservative treatment within 6 weeks, or if time loss extends longer than 2 weeks, specialist consultation should be obtained.

Although botulinum toxin injections of the scalene muscles have been reported to relieve NTOS symptoms,[18] results of a high-quality randomized trial showed no clear clinical improvement related to this treatment.[19] In addition, it seems that there are substantial technical challenges and potentially severe adverse effects from this procedure. Therefore, Botox injections conducted as a diagnostic tool or for treatment of NTOS is not authorized.

When feasible, job modifications that reduce the intensity of manual tasks may prevent progression and promote recovery from NTOS.[17] If symptoms persist despite appropriate treatment, permanent job modifications may still allow patients to remain at work. Patients do not usually need time off from work activities prior to surgery, unless they present with objective weakness or sensory loss in the upper extremity that limits work activities or poses a substantial safety risk.

Surgical Treatment

Surgical treatment of NTOS has been described in narrative reviews, case reports, and retrospective case series.[5,20–35] A population-based study among injured workers in Washington State showed poor outcomes in the majority of cases and significant adverse events in up to 20% of cases.[35] More recent administrative data from Washington State showed similar poor outcomes and far greater expense and disability among TOS cases who received surgery.[36] TOS was on average the 10th diagnosis in cases, indicating that surgery is often requested late in the course of an injured worker's condition, after many other often invasive treatments have failed. TOS surgery should include exploration of the brachial plexus throughout its course in the thoracic outlet to decompress it by resecting any compressive and/or constrictive structures. These may include any of the 3 sites of compression (discussed previously). No specific method of surgical treatment has proved most effective.

Surgical treatment should only be considered if

1. The patient has met the diagnostic criteria (discussed previously) and
2. The condition interferes with work or activities of daily living and
3. The condition does not improve despite conservative treatment

Without confirmation of NTOS by both objective clinical findings and abnormal EDSs, surgery is not authorized.

RETURN TO WORK
Early Assessment

Timeliness of the diagnosis can be a critical factor influencing RTW. Among workers with upper extremity disorders, 7% of workers account for 75% of the long-term disability.[37] A large prospective study in the Washington State workers' compensation system identified several important predictors of long-term disability: low expectations of RTW, no offer of a job accommodation, and high physical demands on the job.[38] Identifying and attending to these risk factors when patients have not returned to work within 2 to 3 weeks of the initial clinical presentation may improve their chances of RTW.

Washington State workers diagnosed accurately and early were far more likely to RTW than workers whose conditions were diagnosed weeks or months later. Early

Table 1
Occupational health quality indicators for neurogenic thoracic outlet syndrome

Clinical Care Action	Time Frame[a]
1. Identify physical stressors from both work and nonwork activities 2. Screen for presence of NTOS 3. Determine work-relatedness 4. Recommend ergonomic improvements or other appropriate job modifications	First health care visit
Communicate with employer regarding RTW using 1. Activity prescription form (or comparable RTW form) and/or 2. Phone call to employer	Each visit while work restrictions exist
1. Assess impediments for RTW 2. Request specialist consultation	If >2 wk of time loss occurs or if there is no clinical improvement within 6 wk of conservative treatment
Specialist consultation	Performed as soon as possible, within 3 wk of request
EDSs	If a diagnosis of NTOS is being considered, schedule studies immediately. These tests are required if time loss extends beyond 2 wk or if surgery is requested.
Surgical decompression	Performed as soon as possible, within 4–6 wk of determining need for surgery

[a] "Time frame" is anchored in time from first provider visit related to NTOS symptoms.

coordination of care with improved timeliness and effective communication with the workplace is also likely to help prevent long-term disability.

A recent quality improvement project in Washington State has demonstrated that delivering medical care according to occupational health best practices similar to those listed in **Table 1** can substantially prevent long-term disability. Findings can be viewed at http://www.lni.wa.gov/ClaimsIns/Providers/ProjResearchComm/OHS/default.asp.

Returning to Work After Surgery

How soon a patient can RTW depends on the type of surgery performed and when rehabilitation begins. Most patients can return to light duty work within 4 to 6 weeks and regular duty within 10 to 12 weeks of surgery.

ELECTRODIAGNOSTIC WORKSHEET

Claim Number: _____

Claimant Name: _____

PURPOSE AND INSTRUCTIONS

The purpose of this worksheet is to help interpret EDSs done for an injured worker. The worksheet should be used only when the main purpose of the study is to evaluate NTOS. It should accompany but not replace the detailed report normally submitted to the insurer.

Electrodiagnostic Worksheet for Work-Related Neurogenic Thoracic Outlet Syndrome

Electrodiagnostic Criteria for Work-Related NTOS Are Met if All Four Boxes Are "Yes"	Check the Correct Box	
	Yes	No
1. Ulnar SNAP[a] <12 uV or absent? OR MABC SNAP[a] amplitude <10 uV or absent, with normal amplitude of the MABC SNAP[a] in the contralateral (unaffected) extremity?		
AND		
2. Median nerve CMAP amplitude <5 mV or absent? OR Ulnar F wave (with or without abnormalities of the median F wave) minimum latency >33 ms or absent, with normal F waves in the contralateral (unaffected) upper extremity? OR Needle EMG showing denervation (eg, fibrillation potentials, positive sharp waves) in at least 1 muscle supplied by each of 2 different nerves from the lower trunk of the brachial plexus, with normal EMG of the cervical paraspinal muscles and at least 1 muscle supplied by a nerve from the middle or upper trunk of the brachial plexus?		
AND		
3. Normal amplitude (≥15 uV) of the median nerve SNAP[a]?		
AND		
4. Normal conduction velocity (≥50 m/s) of the ulnar motor nerve across the elbow?		

[a]Antidromic

Additional Comments:

_____

_____

_____   _____

Signed   Date

GUIDELINE SUMMARY

Review Criteria for the Diagnosis and Treatment of Work-Related Neurogenic Thoracic Outlet Syndrome

CLINICAL FINDINGS				
SUBJECTIVE (Symptoms)	OBJECTIVE (Signs)	DIAGNOSTIC	CONSERVATIVE TREATMENT	SURGICAL TREATMENT
AND				
Pain, paresthesias, or weakness affecting the upper extremity (most commonly affecting the ring or small finger)	AND Tenderness Scalene Trapezius Anterior chest wall Brachial plexus Weakness Loss of finger dexterity Atrophy	EDSs are required to objectively confirm the diagnosis of NTOS. EDS criteria are as follows: 1. Absent or reduced amplitude (<12 uV) of the ulnar SNAP OR Absent or reduced amplitude (<10 uV) of the MABC SNAP with normal amplitude of the MABC SNAP in the contralateral (unaffected) extremity AND 2. Absent or reduced amplitude (<5 mV) of the median CMAP OR Absent or prolonged minimum latency (>33 ms) of the ulnar F wave (with or without abnormalities of the median F wave), and with normal F waves in the contralateral (unaffected) upper extremity OR Needle EMG showing denervation (eg, fibrillation potentials, positive sharp waves) in at least 1 muscle supplied by each of 2 different nerves from the lower trunk of the brachial plexus, with normal EMG of the cervical paraspinal muscles and at least 1 muscle supplied by a nerve from the middle or upper trunk of the brachial plexus AND 3. Normal amplitude (≥15 uV) of the median nerve SNAP AND 4. Normal conduction velocity (≥50 m/s) of the ulnar motor nerve across the elbow	Modify job activities that exacerbate symptoms AND/OR Physical therapy with strengthening and stretching, postural exercises AND/OR Antiinflammatory drug therapy	Surgical treatment should only be considered if 1. The patient has met the diagnostic criteria under the section making the diagnosis AND 2. The condition interferes with work or activities of daily living AND 3. The condition does not improve despite conservative treatment Without confirmation of brachial plexus compression **by both objective clinical findings and abnormal EDSs**, surgery is not authorized.

ACKNOWLEDGMENTS

Acknowledgment and gratitude go to all subcommittee members, clinical experts, and consultants who contributed to this important guideline:

IIMAC members: Gregory T. Carter, MD, MS—Chair; Dianna Chamblin, MD; G.A. DeAndrea, MD, MBA; Jordan Firestone, MD, PhD, MPH; Andrew Friedman, MD; Walter Franklin Krengel III, MD; and Robert G.R. Lang, MD.

Subcommittee clinical experts: Michel Kliot, MD; Mark H. Meissner, MD; Lawrence R. Robinson, MD; Thomas E. Trumble, MD; and Michael D. Weiss, MD.

Consultants: Terrell Kjerulf, MD; and Ken O'Bara, MD.

Department staff who helped develop and prepare this guideline include Gary M. Franklin, MD, MPH, Medical Director; Lee Glass, MD, JD, Associate Medical Director; Simone P. Javaher, BSN, MPA, Occupational Nurse Consultant; and Reshma N. Kearney, MPH, Epidemiologist.

REFERENCES

1. Gronseth GS, Woodroffe LM, Getchius TSD. Clinical Practice Guideline Process Manual. American Academy of Neurology 2011. Available at: http://tools.aan.com/globals/axon/assets/9023.pdf. Accessed May 29, 2015.
2. Watson LA, Pizzari T, Balster S. Thoracic outlet syndrome part 1: clinical manifestations, differentiation, and treatment pathways. Man Ther 2009;14:586–95 Narrative Review.
3. Sanders RJ, Hammond SL. Etiology and pathology. Hand Clin 2004;20(1):23–6 Narrative Review.
4. Pascarelli EF, Hsu YP. Understanding work-related upper extremity disorders: clinical findings in 485 computer users, musicians, and others. J Occup Rehabil 2001;11(1):1–21, IV.
5. Landry GJ, Moneta GL, Taylor LM Jr, et al. Long-term functional outcome of neurogenic thoracic outlet syndrome in surgically and conservatively treated patients. J Vasc Surg 2001;33(2):312–7 [discussion: 317–9]. IV.
6. Brantigan CO, Roos DB. Diagnosing thoracic outlet syndrome. Hand Clin 2004; 20:27–36 Narrative Review.
7. Nord KM, Kapoor P, Fisher J, et al. False positive rate of thoracic outlet syndrome diagnostic maneuvers. Electromyogr Clin Neurophysiol 2008;48(2):67–74, III.
8. Seror P. Symptoms of thoracic outlet syndrome in women with carpal tunnel syndrome. Clin Neurophysiol 2005;116(10):2324–9, IV.
9. Machanic BI, Sanders RJ. Medial antebrachial cutaneous nerve measurements to diagnose neurogenic thoracic outlet syndrome. Ann Vasc Surg 2008;22(2):248–54, III.
10. Seror P. Medial antebrachial cutaneous nerve conduction study, a new tool to demonstrate mild lower brachial plexus lesions. A report of 16 cases. Clin Neurophysiol 2004;115(10):2316–22, IV.
11. Tolson TD. EMG for thoracic outlet syndrome. Hand Clin 2004;20:37–42 Narrative Review.
12. Rousseff R, Tzvetanov P, Valkov I. Utility (or futility?) of electrodiagnosis in thoracic outlet syndrome. Electromyogr Clin Neurophysiol 2005;45(3):131–3, IV.
13. Torriani M, Gupta R, Donahue DM. Sonographically guided anesthetic injection of anterior scalene muscle for investigation of neurogenic thoracic outlet syndrome. Skeletal Radiol 2009;38:1083–7, IV.
14. Jordan SE, Machleder HI. Diagnosis of thoracic outlet syndrome using electrophysiologically guided anterior scalene blocks. Ann Vasc Surg 1998;12(3):260–4, IV.

15. Vanti C, Natalini L, Romeo A, et al. Conservative treatment of thoracic outlet syndrome. Eura Medicophys 2007;43:55–70 Systematic Review.
16. Hanif S, Tassadaq N, Rathore MF, et al. Role of therapeutic exercises in neurogenic thoracic outlet syndrome. J Ayub Med Coll Abbottabad 2007;19(4): 85–8, III.
17. Crosby CA, Wehbe MA. Conservative treatment for thoracic outlet syndrome. Hand Clin 2004;20:43–9 Narrative Review.
18. Jordan SE, Ahn SS, Gelabert HA. Combining ultrasonography and electromyography for botulinum chemodenervation treatment of thoracic outlet syndrome: comparison with fluoroscopy and electromyography guidance. Pain Physician 2007;10(4):541–6, IV.
19. Finlayson HC, O'Connor RJ, Brasher PM, et al. Botulinum toxin injection for management of thoracic outlet syndrome: a double-blind, randomized, controlled trial. Pain 2011;152:2023–8, I.
20. Povlsen B, Belzberg A, Hansson T, et al. Treatment for thoracic outlet syndrome [review]. Cochrane Database Syst Rev 2010;(1):CD007218. III.
21. Chang DC, Rotellini-Coltvet LA, Mukherjee D, et al. Surgical intervention for thoracic outlet syndrome improves patient's quality of life. J Vasc Surg 2009; 49(3):630–5 [discussion: 635–7]. IV.
22. Chang DC, Lidor AO, Matsen SL, et al. Reported in-hospital complications following rib resections for neurogenic thoracic outlet syndrome. Ann Vasc Surg 2007;21(5):564–70 Observational Study.
23. Abdellaoui A, Atwan M, Reid F, et al. Endoscopic assisted transaxillary first rib resection. Interact Cardiovasc Thorac Surg 2007;6(5):644–6, IV.
24. Colli BO, Carlotti CG Jr, Assirati JA Jr, et al. Neurogenic thoracic outlet syndromes: a comparison of true and nonspecific syndromes after surgical treatment. Surg Neurol 2006;65(3):262–71 [discussion: 271–2]. IV.
25. Krishnan KG, Pinzer T, Schackert G. The transaxillary approach in the treatment of thoracic outlet syndrome: a neurosurgical appraisal. Zentralbl Neurochir 2005; 66(4):180–9, IV.
26. Altobelli GG, Kudo T, Haas BT, et al. Thoracic outlet syndrome: pattern of clinical success after operative decompression. J Vasc Surg 2005;42(1):122–8, IV.
27. Sanders RJ, Hammond SL. Supraclavicular first rib resection and total scalenectomy: technique and results. Hand Clin 2004;20(1):61–70 Narrative Review.
28. Samarasam I, Sadhu D, Agarwal S, et al. Surgical management of thoracic outlet syndrome: a 10-year experience. ANZ J Surg 2004;74(6):450–4, IV.
29. Nannapaneni R, Marks SM. Neurogenic thoracic outlet syndrome. Br J Neurosurg 2003;17(2):144–8, IV.
30. Maxey TS, Reece TB, Ellman PI, et al. Safety and efficacy of the supraclavicular approach to thoracic outlet decompression. Ann Thorac Surg 2003;76(2):396–9 [discussion 399–400]; IV.
31. Bhattacharya V, Hansrani M, Wyatt MG, et al. Outcome following surgery for thoracic outlet syndrome. Eur J Vasc Endovasc Surg 2003;26(2):170–5, IV.
32. Balci AE, Balci TA, Cakir O, et al. Surgical treatment of thoracic outlet syndrome: effect and results of surgery. Ann Thorac Surg 2003;75(4):1091–6 [discussion: 1096]. IV.
33. Sharp WJ, Nowak LR, Zamani T, et al. Long-term follow-up and patient satisfaction after surgery for thoracic outlet syndrome. Ann Vasc Surg 2001; 15(1):32–6, IV.
34. Athanassiadi K, Kalavrouziotis G, Karydakis K, et al. Treatment of thoracic outlet syndrome: long-term results. World J Surg 2001;25(5):553–7, IV.

35. Franklin GM, Fulton-Kehoe D, Bradley C, et al. Outcome of surgery for thoracic outlet syndrome in Washington state workers' compensation. Neurology 2000; 54(6):1252–7, III.
36. Franklin GM. Workers' compensation issues in thoracic outlet syndrome. In: Illig KA, Thompson RW, Freischlag JA, et al, editors. Thoracic outlet syndrome. New York: Springer; 2012. IV.
37. Hashemi L, Webster B, Clance E, et al. Length of disability and cost of work-related musculoskeletal disorders of the upper extremity. J Occup Environ Med 1998;40:261–9, III.
38. Turner J, Franklin G, Fulton-Kehoe D. Early predictors of chronic work disability associated with carpal tunnel syndrome: a longitudinal workers' compensation cohort study. Am J Ind Med 2007;50:489–500, I.

Work-Related Complex Regional Pain Syndrome

Diagnosis and Treatment

Andrew Friedman, MD[a,b]

KEYWORDS

- Complex regional pain syndrome • RSD • Diagnosis • Treatment
- Evidence-based review • Workers compensation

KEY POINTS

- Prevention and early identification of complex regional pain syndrome (CRPS) are critical in regard to optimizing outcomes. Use of vitamin C can be helpful in preventing CRPS in cases of distal extremity injury.
- Risk factors include injury or immobilization of a distal extremity, female sex, fear of movement, and tobacco use. Failure to follow a normal course of return to function should warrant closer attention by the physician.
- The diagnosis of CRPS requires the presence of a specific set of symptoms and findings in addition to pain.
- A phased approach to treatment is presented. CRPS should be identified early and the patient moved quickly to more integrated and experienced levels of care aimed at reactivation if not improving.

INTRODUCTION

This guideline is to be used by physicians, claim managers, occupational nurses, all other providers, and utilization review staff. The emphasis is on accurate diagnosis and treatment that is curative or rehabilitative (see Washington Administrative Code [WAC] 296-20-01,002 for definitions).

This guideline was developed between 2010 and 2011 by the Industrial Insurance Medical Advisory Committee (IIMAC) and its subcommittee on chronic noncancer pain. The subcommittee presented its work to the full IIMAC, and the IIMAC voted with full consensus advising the Washington State Department of Labor & Industries to adopt the guideline. This guideline is based on the best available clinical and scientific evidence from a systematic review of the literature and a consensus of expert

[a] Department of Physical Medicine and Rehabilitation, University of WA, 1410 NE Campus Parkway, WA 98195, USA; [b] Virginia Mason Medical Center, 1100 9th Avenue, Seattle, WA 98111, USA
E-mail address: andrew.friedman.001@gmail.com

Phys Med Rehabil Clin N Am 26 (2015) 563–572
http://dx.doi.org/10.1016/j.pmr.2015.04.006
1047-9651/15/$ – see front matter © 2015 Elsevier Inc. All rights reserved.

opinion. One of the committee's primary goals is to provide standards that ensure high quality of care for injured workers in Washington State.

Complex regional pain syndrome (CRPS), sometimes referred to as reflex sympathetic dystrophy or causalgia, is an uncommon chronic condition with clinical features that include pain, sensory, sudomotor and vasomotor disturbances, trophic changes, and impaired motor function.[1–3] This condition may involve the upper or lower extremities and can affect men or women of any age, race, or ethnicity. Most people with onset of CRPS are females and adults. Females are affected as least 3 times more than males.[2,3] The pathophysiology of CRPS is not fully understood. When CRPS occurs it typically follows an injury, such as a fracture, sprain, crush injury, or surgery.[4,5] Immobilization, particularly after fracture or surgery, is a well-described risk factor.[5,6]

Two types of CRPS have been described: CRPS I and CRPS II. For the most part, the clinical characteristics of both types are the same. The difference is based on the presence or absence of nerve damage. CRPS I (also known as reflex sympathetic dystrophy) is not associated with nerve damage, whereas CRPS II (also known as causalgia) is associated with objective evidence of nerve damage. Treatment for either form of CRPS should follow the recommendations in this guideline, although if there is objective evidence for CRPS II, other references and treatment guidelines for the particular nerve injury may also apply.

ESTABLISHING WORK RELATEDNESS

CRPS may occur as a delayed complication of a work-related condition or its treatment.[4,5] Usually, CRPS occurs following an injury. In rare situations, CRPS may occur following an occupational disease. An injury is defined as a sudden and tangible happening of a traumatic nature producing an immediate or prompt result and occurring from without. The only requirement for establishing work-relatedness for an injury is that it occurs in the course of employment.

For an occupational disease, establishing work relatedness requires a more critical analysis that demonstrates more than a simple association between the disease and workplace activities. Establishing work relatedness for an occupational disease requires

1. Exposure: workplace activities that contribute to or cause the condition
2. Outcome: a medical condition that meets certain diagnostic criteria
3. Relationship: generally accepted scientific evidence that establishes on a more probable than not basis (greater than 50%) that the workplace activity (exposure) in an individual case was a proximate cause of the development or worsening of the condition (outcome)

Establishing CRPS as a work-related condition requires documentation of

1. Another work-related condition has been previously accepted
2. A diagnosis of CRPS that meets the criteria in further section
3. CRPS involves the same body part as the accepted, work-related condition

PREVENTION

CRPS is believed to be incited by trauma or immobilization following trauma. It is most likely to occur in the setting of bone fracture, especially of the distal extremity. The greatest risk for CRPS appears to be certain types of fractures such as distal radial, tibial, and ankle, as well as limited movement of the affected limb.[6–9]

CRPS may be preventable if the alert clinician is on the lookout for CRPS. Therefore, in addition to the usual protocols for a particular injury, close surveillance of patients at risk for CRPS is recommended. For such patients, extra office visits may be appropriate, especially if the clinician suspects a patient may not follow the expected course of recovery within the expected length of time. The use of vitamin C (500 mg by mouth every day for 50 days) has been shown to reduce the incidence of CRPS following radial, foot, and ankle fractures (based on Level I and Level II Evidence).[8,9]

CRPS may be prevented or arrested by early identification of risk factors and taking prompt action when they are present. The emphasis should be on pain control, mobilization, and monitoring from onset of acute injury through the normally expected treatment time, typically a few weeks to a few months.

To help prevent CRPS, one should know the risk factors and identify cases early and take action.

Know the Risk Factors

Risk factors include

1. Prolonged immobilization (eg, due to bone fractures or soft tissue injury, especially in upper or lower distal extremities)
2. Longer than normal healing times
3. Delays in reactivation after immobility (eg, due to inadequate control of acute pain)
4. Lack of weight bearing on lower extremities
5. Tobacco use, which can delay fracture healing
6. Reluctance to move or reactivate because of fear of pain or injury (fear avoidance)
7. Nerve damage

Identify Cases Early and Take Action

One should take the following steps

1. Intentionally solicit symptoms and watch for signs
2. Educate the patient to immediately report any CRPS symptoms
3. Give clear and specific instructions to patients about mobilization and use of the injured part
4. Manage patients' expectations about pain relief
5. Use vitamin C at recommended doses in cases of fracture

Encourage Active Participation in Rehabilitation

One should take the following actions

1. Have patient keep a recovery diary, logging pain level, symptoms, and activities
2. Provide or facilitate activity coaching
3. Set recovery goals with specified time frames (eg, next office or physical therapy visit)
4. Use medications or interventional procedures in concert with rehabilitative strategies

MAKING THE DIAGNOSIS

Most patients with pain in an extremity do not have CRPS. Avoid the mistake of diagnosing CRPS primarily because a patient has widespread extremity pain that does not fit an obvious anatomic pattern. In many instances, there is no diagnostic label that adequately describes the patient's symptoms. It is often more appropriate to describe the condition as regional pain of undetermined origin than to diagnose CRPS. However, it is equally important to identify CRPS when it does occur, so that appropriate treatment can be instituted.

Symptoms and Signs

CRPS is an uncommon syndrome based on a particular pattern of symptoms and signs in addition to pain.[2,3] Symptoms and signs may be present at rest or elicited by exercise or activity involving the affected limb. The primary symptom associated with CRPS is continuous pain that is disproportionate to the inciting event.[10] Pain is often described as burning or sharp and may be associated with changes in skin sensation such as hyperalgesia (increased sensitivity) or allodynia (pain perception to stimuli that are normally not painful). Other symptoms and signs in the affected area may include

1. Skin temperature dysregulation
2. Skin color variability
3. Sweat dysregulation
4. Swelling or edema
5. Changes to the texture or growth pattern of hair, nails, or skin
6. Motor weakness, decreased range of motion (ROM), tremors, or dystonia

Three-Phase Bone Scintigraphy

Three-phase bone scintigraphy can be a useful supplement to making the clinical diagnosis of CRPS (Based on Level II and Level IV evidence).[11,12] Abnormalities related to CRPS that may be seen in a 3-phase bone scan include increased blood flow and increased blood pool uptake to the region of interest, with delayed images showing increased uptake in a periarticular pattern. Including the bone scan as a criterion is intended to increase diagnostic sensitivity. A normal bone scan neither increases nor decreases the likelihood of the diagnosis of CRPS. An abnormal bone scan is not required for a CRPS diagnosis.

Diagnostic Criteria

Diagnostic criteria for CRPS, known as the Budapest criteria, were adopted by the subcommittee, with slight modification, after careful consideration of existing criteria and available scientific evidence. Information about the sensitivity and specificity of the diagnostic signs and symptoms can be found in the literature (**Box 1**).[13–15]

TREATMENT
Have a Treatment Plan

Treatment for CRPS should be initiated early and aggressively. An interdisciplinary approach is often useful. A treatment plan should encourage patients to take an active role in their rehabilitation plan. This can include having the patient keep a journal, to record symptoms, activity tolerance, and pain and function levels. Emphasis should be on improving functional activity in the symptomatic limb and should include elements of the following

- Physical therapy or occupational therapy
- Medication for pain control
- Psychological or psychiatric consultation and therapy
- Sympathetic blocks
- Multidisciplinary program for pain management

Physical and occupational therapy
A physical or occupational therapy treatment plan specific to CRPS should be developed by a therapist who is experienced in the treatment of CRPS. Therapy should be

> **Box 1**
> **Diagnostic criteria for complex regional pain syndrome**
>
> *To make a clinical diagnosis, the patient must meet all of the following criteria*
>
> 1. Continuing pain, which is disproportionate to any inciting event
> 2. At least one symptom in three of the four following categories must be reported
>   - Sensory: reports of hyperalgesia and/or allodynia (to pinprick, light touch, deep somatic pressure, and/or joint movement)
>   - Vasomotor: reports of instability and/or asymmetry of skin temperature and/or color
>   - Sudomotor/edema: reports of instability and/or asymmetry of sweating and/or edema
>   - Motor/trophic: reports of decreased range of motion and/or motor dysfunction (eg, weakness, tremor, or dystonia) and/or trophic changes (eg, hair, nails, or skin)
> 3. At least one sign in two or more of the following categories must be identified by objective clinical findings documented in the medical record over the course of one or more examinations (a 3-phase bone scan that is abnormal in a pattern characteristic of CRPS can be substituted for one of the signs in this section [this is the committee's modification of the Budapest criteria])
>   - Sensory: evidence of hyperalgesia and/or allodynia (to pinprick, light touch, deep somatic pressure, and/or joint movement)
>   - Vasomotor: evidence of instability and/or asymmetry of skin temperature and/or color
>   - Sudomotor/edema: evidence of instability and/or asymmetry of sweating and/or edema
>   - Motor/trophic: evidence of decreased range of motion and/or motor dysfunction (eg, weakness, tremor, or dystonia) and/or trophic changes (eg, hair, nails, or skin)
> 4. There is no other diagnosis that better explains the signs and symptoms

active, focused on desensitization, normalizing movement patterns, improving strength and range of motion, and improving functional activities. A CRPS- focused physical or occupational therapy plan should include the following elements:

A. An evaluation to include:
   1. Date of onset of original injury (helpful in determining if early or late stage) and a date of onset of the CRPS symptoms and signs
   2. Baseline objective measurements including range of motion of all involved joints, strength, sensory loss, hypersensitivity, appearance, temperature, function (eg, weight bearing and gait for lower extremity; fine motor tasks, pinch, and grip for upper extremity), and use of assistive devices, braces, and orthotics; if possible, include objective measurements of swelling
B. Specific, measurable functional goals that will allow assessment of progress and the effectiveness of treatment for the affected area
C. All treatment programs should include a core of
   1. Desensitization
   2. Neuromuscular re-education, which might include graded motor imagery,[16,17] mirror box therapy,[18] or other techniques to promote normalization of neuromuscular function (based on Level II evidence)
   3. A progressive, active exercise program designed to promote improvement in range of motion, strength, and endurance
   4. Activities targeted to attain the functional goals, eg, weight bearing and gait training for the lower extremity and fine motor tasks for the upper extremity

5. A monitored home exercise program to promote the patient's participation in rehabilitation activities on a daily basis

D. Documentation should be done at least every 2 weeks to include
1. Reassessment of relevant baseline measurements described previously; this provides objective evidence of response or nonresponse to treatment
2. Assessment of progress toward functional goals (eg, how the condition interferes with daily activities or activities related to employment)
3. Level of patient motivation
4. Participation in a home exercise program

Medication for pain control

Pain inhibits movement, and inadequate pain control may be an obstacle to activity, so judicious use of medications for pain control can be a useful adjunct to therapy. There is no drug with high-quality evidence to support use in either pain reduction or facilitation of function in CRPS. However, the committee recognizes that various medications are commonly used in clinical practice to manage pain or associated symptoms in CRPS.[19] The categories of medications often used include nonsteroidal anti-inflammatory drugs (NSAIDs), anticonvulsants,[20] antidepressants, opioids, N-methyl-D-aspartate receptor antagonists (NMDAs), antihypertensives, alpha-adrenergic agents, calcitonin,[21] and bisphosphonates.[22] Selection of a particular agent may be influenced by the specific symptom or associated comorbidities. These medications may be useful in helping a patient engage in therapy and regain function—the keys to successful management of CRPS.

The benefits of pain control should be weighed against the risks associated with adverse effects. This is a particular challenge when using opioid medications for chronic pain. For further detail about this challenging topic, refer to the article in this volume on opioid prescribing in the workers compensation environment. The Guideline on Opioid Dosing for Chronic Non-Cancer Pain, developed by the Washington State Agency Medical Directors Group can also help: http://www.agencymeddirectors.wa. gov/Files/OpioidGdline.pdf.

Psychological or psychiatric consultation and therapy

It is not uncommon for a fear-avoidance behavior pattern to emerge with a CRPS diagnosis. Patients are frequently fearful that pain indicates danger. They are sometimes concerned that ongoing pain means their condition has been misdiagnosed. Consequently, education and frequent reassurance are essential.

This may be addressed using cognitive–behavioral therapy. In many cases, there is a more substantial psychological barrier to using the limb that warrants direct attention. If a comorbid mental illness is identified that warrants formal psychiatric evaluation and treatment, screening or referral to the appropriate specialist may be needed.

Sympathetic blocks

Sympathetic blocks have long been a standard treatment for CRPS and can be useful for a subset of cases. Stellate ganglion blocks (cervical sympathetic blocks) and lumbar sympathetic blocks are widely used in the management of upper and lower extremity CRPS. There is limited evidence to confirm effectiveness.[23] An initial trial of up to 3 sympathetic blocks should be considered when the condition fails to improve with conservative treatment, including analgesia and physical therapy.

The most common way to administer sympathetic blocks is a single local anesthetic injection. Selection of sympathetic block technique depends on each case, reflecting in part the patient's needs and the interventional pain specialist's preference and expertise. The current standard of practice is to use image-guided approaches, such as with fluoroscopy and ultrasound, since complications of blind injections may include airway hematomas, inadvertent intravascular or central neuraxial injections and esophageal puncture. Sympathetic blocks done without imaging guidance will not be authorized.

When sympathetic blocks are helpful, the benefit is evident within the first days following the nerve block. The optimal timing, number, or frequency of blocks, have not been specified. Patients who have a shorter duration of symptoms seem to have a greater response to treatment.[24,25] Documentation of a physiologic response (eg, change in skin temperature of the affected limb or Horner syndrome) is required to demonstrate that the block was successful. For sympathetic blocks to support lasting improvement, they should be combined with physical and behavioral therapies. Therapy should occur within 24 hours of the block or, if possible, on the same day of the block. An effective block is expected to produce at least 50% improvement in pain and a concomitant increase in function. Sympathetic blocks may be repeated, only when there is objective evidence of progressive improvement in pain and function.

Multidisciplinary treatment

A multidisciplinary program for pain management will provide coordinated and closely monitored care using physical and/or occupational therapy, medication management, psychological screening and counseling, patient education, and other pain management techniques. The goal is to coordinate therapeutic interventions that ensure adequate pain control so reactivation of the affected body part can occur. It is recommended that the attending provider and the pain management team communicate regularly about the patient's treatment plan and progress toward treatment goals. Therapists and pain management staff should routinely report objective and quantifiable measures of functional improvement and pain tolerance and alert the attending provider if progress is not occurring. The objective is to act quickly so that the treatment team may take actions to quickly get the patient back on the expected course of recovery.

Treatment in Phases

Treatment can be thought of in phases. Although each phase has a general time frame, the time needed for an individual case is difficult to predict. Each phase can be shortened or lengthened as needed, allowing patients to move from 1 phase to another depending on their individual progress.

Phase one—prevention and mitigation of complex regional pain syndrome risk factors

The duration of Phase One will depend on the expected healing time for the specific injury, commonly spanning the first few weeks following the injury. The emphasis during Phase One is on pain control, appropriate mobilization, and monitoring of pain and function. After an initial injury, the patient should be encouraged to move as much as is safe for whatever injury he or she has. Physical therapy and occupational therapy will be directed at what is appropriate for the specific injury and may be limited during this phase. Although there are no fixed rules as to the time of immobilization for a given injury, 6 to 8 weeks for the upper extremity and 8 to 12 weeks for the lower extremity are typical durations. It may be worth noting that mobility can continue in spite of casting. For example, a patient in a long arm cast can still move his or her fingers, and a patient in an ankle cast can still move his or her toes. With appropriate immobilization, pain should generally decrease progressively with time. If pain is not decreasing over time, the provider must reassess the plan of treatment. If at any point the patient demonstrates unusual distress, pain complaints that appear to be out of proportion to the injury, or unexpectedly slow progress, the frequency of clinic visits should be increased. In this situation, it is important to consider the possibility of a missed diagnosis or an unrecognized comorbidity such as a behavioral or substance abuse disorder.

Phase two—recovery is not normal
The sooner treatment for suspected CRPS is initiated, the more likely it is that the long-term outcome will be good. When recovery is delayed, and if no specific cause for the delay is identified, CRPS may be the diagnosis. Referral to a pain management or rehabilitation medicine specialist is strongly recommended.

Phase three—complex regional pain syndrome initial treatment
Following a CRPS diagnosis, treatment should be initiated early and aggressively in the patient's community whenever possible. Care should be coordinated and include physical or occupational therapy, psychological or psychiatric therapy, and medication management. An initial sympathetic block trial may be considered in cases that do not demonstrate functional gains during initial treatment.

Phase four—complex regional pain syndrome intensive treatment
When the patient is unlikely to benefit from Phase Three treatment, an immediate referral to a multidisciplinary treatment program may be made. If the patient's condition has not substantially improved within 6 weeks of Phase Three treatment, referral to an approved multidisciplinary treatment program is recommended.

Treatment not authorized for complex regional pain syndrome
The following interventions are not authorized for CRPS

- Sympathectomy (no effect/no improvement in function[26])
- Spinal cord stimulation (noncovered benefit; see Health Technology Assessment decision 2010; note that Washington State law requires Labor and Industries (L&I) to follow decisions made by the Health technology assessment (HTA) (http://www.hta.hca.wa.gov/documents/adopted_findings_decision_scs_102510.pdf)
- Ketamine infusions (no effect/no improvement in function, serious adverse events (based on Level II evidence).[27,28]

ACKNOWLEDGMENTS

Acknowledgment and gratitude go to all subcommittee members, clinical experts, and consultants who contributed to this important guideline: IIMAC committee members Ruth Bishop, MD, A. Friedman, MD – Chair, Jordan Firestone, MD, PhD, MPH, David Tauben, MD, Gerald Yorioka, MD; subcommittee clinical experts Ray Baker, MD, Heather Kroll, MD, Jim Robinson, MD, Irakli Soulakvelidze, MD, Wyndam Strodtbeck, MD; consultants Ken O'Bara MD, Roger Allen, PhD, PT, Department staff who helped develop and prepare this guideline include: Gary M. Franklin, MD, MPH, Medical Director, Lee Glass, MD, JD, Associate Medical Director, Simone P. Javaher, BSN, MPA, Occupational Nurse Consultant, Reshma N. Kearney, MPH, Epidemiologist, Hal Stockbridge, MD, MPH, Associate Medical Director.

REFERENCES

1. Harden R, Bruehl S. Diagnosis of complex regional pain syndrome: signs, symptoms, and new empirically derived diagnostic criteria. Clin J Pain 2006;22(5): 415–9.

2. de Mos M, de Bruijn AG, Huygen FJ, et al. The incidence of complex regional pain syndrome: a population-based study. Pain 2007;129(1–2):12–20.
3. Sandroni P, Benrud-Larson LM, McClelland RL, et al. Complex regional pain syndrome type I: incidence and prevalence in Olmsted county, a population-based study. Pain 2003;103(1–2):199–207.
4. Duman I, Dincer U, Taskaynatan MA, et al. Reflex sympathetic dystrophy: a retrospective epidemiological study of 168 patients. Clin Rheumatol 2007;26(9): 1433–7.
5. Allen G, Galer BS, Schwartz L. Epidemiology of complex regional pain syndrome: a retrospective chart review of 134 patients. Pain 1999;80(3):539–44.
6. Terkelsen AJ, Bach FW, Jensen TS. Experimental forearm immobilization in humans induces cold and mechanical hyperalgesia. Anesthesiology 2008; 109(2):297–307.
7. Besse JL, Gadeyne S, Galand-Desme S, et al. Effect of vitamin C on prevention of complex regional pain syndrome type I in foot and ankle surgery. Foot Ankle Surg 2009;15(4):179–82.
8. Zollinger PE, Tuinebreijer WE, Breederveld RS, et al. Can vitamin C prevent complex regional pain syndrome in patients with wrist fractures? A randomized, controlled, multicenter dose-response study. J Bone Joint Surg Am 2007;89(7): 1424–31.
9. Zollinger PE, Tuinebreijer WE, Kreis RW, et al. Effect of vitamin C on frequency of reflex sympathetic dystrophy in wrist fractures: a randomised trial. Lancet 1999; 354(9195):2025–8.
10. Stanton-Hicks M. Complex regional pain syndrome. Anesthesiol Clin North America 2003;21:733–44.
11. Wuppenhorst N, Maier C, Frettloh J, et al. Sensitivity and specificity of 3-phase bone scintigraphy in the diagnosis of complex regional pain syndrome of the upper extremity. Clin J Pain 2010;26(3):182–9.
12. Zyluk A. The usefulness of quantitative evaluation of three-phase scintigraphy in the diagnosis of post-traumatic reflex sympathetic dystrophy. J Hand Surg Br 1999;24(1):16–21.
13. Harden RN, Bruehl S, Perez RS, et al. Validation of proposed diagnostic criteria (the "Budapest Criteria") for complex regional pain syndrome. Pain 2010;150(2): 268–74.
14. Bruehl S, Harden RN, Galer BS, et al. External validation of IASP diagnostic criteria for complex regional pain syndrome and proposed research diagnostic criteria. International Association for the Study of Pain. Pain 1999;81(1–2):147–54.
15. Harden RN, Bruehl S, Galer BS, et al. Complex regional pain syndrome: are the IASP diagnostic criteria valid and sufficiently comprehensive? Pain 1999;83(2):211–9.
16. Moseley GL. Graded motor imagery for pathologic pain: a randomized controlled trial. Neurology 2006;67(12):2129–34.
17. Moseley GL. Graded motor imagery is effective for long-standing complex regional pain syndrome: a randomised controlled trial. Pain 2004;108(1–2):192–8.
18. Cacchio A, De Blasis E, De Blasis V, et al. Mirror therapy in complex regional pain syndrome type 1 of the upper limb in stroke patients. Neurorehabil Neural Repair 2009;23(8):792–9.
19. Perez RS, Zollinger PE, Dijkstra PU, et al. Evidence based guidelines for complex regional pain syndrome type 1. BMC Neurol 2010;10:20.
20. van de Vusse AC, Stomp-van den Berg SG, Kessels AH, et al. Randomised controlled trial of gabapentin in Complex Regional Pain Syndrome type 1 [ISRCTN84121379]. BMC Neurol 2004;4:13.

21. Sahin F, Yilmaz F, Kotevoglu N, et al. Efficacy of salmon calcitonin in complex regional pain syndrome (type 1) in addition to physical therapy. Clin Rheumatol 2006;25(2):143–8.
22. Brunner F, Schmid A, Kissling R, et al. Biphosphonates for the therapy of complex regional pain syndrome I–systematic review. Eur J Pain 2009;13(1):17–21.
23. Cepeda MS, Carr DB, Lau J. Local anesthetic sympathetic blockade for complex regional pain syndrome. Cochrane Database Syst Rev 2005;(4):CD004598.
24. Yucel I, Demiraran Y, Ozturan K, et al. Complex regional pain syndrome type I: efficacy of stellate ganglion blockade. J Orthop Traumatol 2009;10(4):179–83.
25. Ackerman WE, Zhang JM. Efficacy of stellate ganglion blockade for the management of type 1 complex regional pain syndrome. South Med J 2006; 99(10):1084–8.
26. Straube S, Derry S, Moore RA, et al. Cervico-thoracic or lumbar sympathectomy for neuropathic pain and complex regional pain syndrome. Cochrane Database Syst Rev 2010;(7):CD002918.
27. Schwartzman RJ, Patel M, Grothusen JR, et al. Efficacy of 5-day continuous lidocaine infusion for the treatment of refractory complex regional pain syndrome. Pain Med 2009;10(2):401–12.
28. Sigtermans MJ, van Hilten JJ, Bauer MC, et al. Ketamine produces effective and long-term pain relief in patients with complex regional pain syndrome Type 1. Pain 2009;145(3):304–11.

Index

Note: Page numbers of article titles are in **boldface** type.

A

AC. *See* Acromioclavicular (AC)
ACDF. *See* Anterior cervical discectomy with fusion (ACDF)
Acromioclavicular (AC) arthritis
    guideline for, 474, 481
    surgery for
        criteria for, 477–478
Acromioclavicular (AC) dislocation
    guideline for, 473
    surgery for
        criteria for, 478
Adjacent segment pathology (ASP), 504–505
Agency executive policy authority, 439–440
Agency regulatory authority, 439
Anterior cervical discectomy with fusion (ACDF), 501
Arthritis
    AC
        guideline for, 474, 481
        surgery for
            criteria for, 477–478
    glenohumeral
        guideline for, 481–482
Arthroscopy
    diagnostic
        guideline for, 482
ASP. *See* Adjacent segment pathology (ASP)
Authority
    agency executive policy, 439–440
    agency regulatory, 439
    statutory, 437–439

B

Biceps
    long head of
        tendinopathy of
            guideline for, 481
Biceps instability
    surgery for
        criteria for, 479

Phys Med Rehabil Clin N Am 26 (2015) 573–581
http://dx.doi.org/10.1016/S1047-9651(15)00061-3
1047-9651/15/$ – see front matter © 2015 Elsevier Inc. All rights reserved.

pmr.theclinics.com

Moving?

Make sure your subscription moves with you!

To notify us of your new address, find your **Clinics Account Number** (located on your mailing label above your name), and contact customer service at:

Email: journalscustomerservice-usa@elsevier.com

800-654-2452 (subscribers in the U.S. & Canada)
314-447-8871 (subscribers outside of the U.S. & Canada)

Fax number: 314-447-8029

Elsevier Health Sciences Division
Subscription Customer Service
3251 Riverport Lane
Maryland Heights, MO 63043

ELSEVIER

Printed and bound by CPI Group (UK) Ltd, Croydon, CR0 4YY

03/10/2024

01040489-0016